Children of Promise

The Parent's Ultimate Guide to Healthy, Happy and Inspired Children

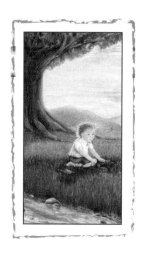

Skyward Publishing

© 2005 by Skyward Publishing
info@skywardpublishing.com

Library of Congress Cataloging-in-Publication Data

Olson, Rand.
  Children of promise : the parent's ultimate guide to healthy, happy, and inspired children / Rand Olson.
      p. cm.
   ISBN 978-1-881554-44-9
  1. Child rearing. 2. Parenting. 3. Children--Health and hygiene. 4.
Family--Health and hygiene. 5. Self-actualization (Psychology)
I. Title.

HQ769.O52 2005
649'.1--dc22

2005002220

Cover illustration by Casey Frisch
Cover and page design by Angela Donelle Underwood
www.coverdiva.com

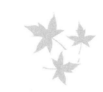

CONTENTS

Prologue

My talent, God given and not of my own design, is to see to the bottom of the real issues of life. This book is a compilation of my experiences accumulated through tens of thousands of visits with patients who are stressed in one or more aspect of their life. Uncontrolled stress will eventually affect health, and health is a vital part of this book. To begin this extraordinary learning opportunity together, we should have the same understanding on a couple of issues. Let's start with a clear understanding of what we mean by the term "health." Health is the ability to be fully and consciously aware of all that contributes to your life experience and to effectively exist in that environment. It then means you see yourself as you really are.

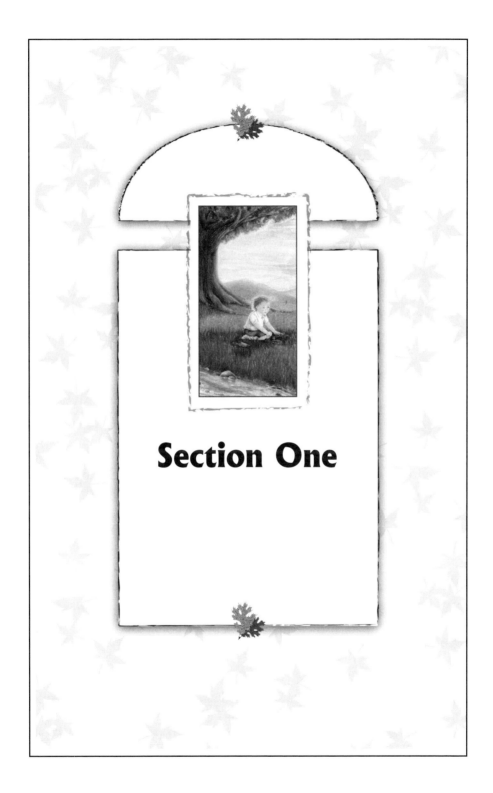

Section One

Chapter 1
The Most Sacred Trust

*To love deeply in one direction makes us
more loving in all others.*
—Anne-Sophie Swetchine

One of the most sacred trusts we have in life is the trust God places in us to nurture the seeds of divinity we call children. The ultimate objective in parenthood is to love our children, teach them correct principles, and give them what they need to become all they can become. We walk daily with the incredible charge to set the foundation on which our children will build their mortal and eternal palace. As we teach them correct principles by word and deed, we are helping to set a solid platform on which they will live their lives.

The Most Sacred Gift
Among the most sacred gifts you can give your child is the gift of health. This gift is best given by example, so create that state in your own life first. Health, if present, allows our dreams and possibilities to become realities. Without health, our potential in life will be limited. Health expands our perception to the

limits of our vast God-given potential. As we mature and develop awareness to match our potential, our ability to enjoy full health is realized. As our health improves, it increases our awareness to allow our potential to blossom and create the fruit of abundance in our lives. As we enjoy this fruit, we sow the seeds of greatness in our children. They will, in turn, have the chance to do the same in their lives.

Harness the Full Expression of Health

Some children are born with great physical challenges. For these special children, the idea of perfect physical health is not a reality, but there is nothing of enduring goodness they cannot find in their given condition. They can still pursue optimal health, despite their circumstances and according to their potential. Health is not a physical accomplishment but the manifestation of our awareness of who we are and integrity in living out of that knowledge. True health broadens our perspectives to enable us to see beyond mortality into our eternal actualities. There is no physical limitation that can harness the full expression of health at this spiritual level of reality.

While some children may have a physical handicap, the nature of life, as it has been divinely ordered, will allow that child to express him or herself in other ways. This expression allows maximal freedom, power, joy, and love to be present in a parent's life and their children's lives.

Chapter 2
Be, Do, and Have: The Three Motives

*Level with your child by being honest. Nobody spots a
phony quicker than a child.*
—Mary MacCracken

There is a foundational idea that when understood brings great insight. There are three motivations in life: the motivations to have, to do, and to be. If we think we need to have different ingredients in our lives, we will always lack in our appreciation and experience in life. Some people think: If I just had a better car, then I would be popular. If I just had better hair, prettier eyes, or better teeth, I could be happy. Some people believe a better job will make them happier or that more money will solve all their problems. To focus on having more of anything will never change our lives in any substantial way. More money will only bring more (similar) existing problems. More of anything only makes us more of what we already are. If we are happy, it can bring more happiness. If we are depressed, it will make us more depressed.

If we focus our efforts on doing, we will always fall short of our real potential. We can set goals and work on changing behaviors and actions, but until we change our intentions, nothing will really change in our inner lives. We can do all the right things, but if we do not do them for the right reasons, they will never have the power to change our internal view of life.

The highest level of perception is the focus on being. This focus gives us full motivation to take complete responsibility for how we feel. It gives us power to choose how we view every situation. By focusing on being, we will automatically begin to do the best of which we are capable. By being our best, we automatically work under the umbrella of integrity and a pure intention. By becoming our best, we will naturally have anything we choose. As we become all that we have the capacity to become, we will have healthy wants, desires, and actions.

Focusing on being allows our real potential to be displayed. We will come to recognize we are incredible the way we are. We will begin to see our true potential. In every situation, it is important to start by being aware in life of what level you are focusing on: having, doing, or being.

Chapter 3
The Big Rocks: Do You Know Yours?

*He who postpones the hour of living is like the rustic who
waits for the river to run out before he crosses it."*
—Horace

The story is told of a man teaching a class one day. He
stood behind his desk. He set a large glass jar on top of the desk
and filled it with large rocks. When it was completely full, he
asked the class: "Is the jar full?" The class responded, "Yes, it is
full." He then picked up a container of gravel from behind the
desk and proceeded to fill the jar with gravel. He sifted the gravel into the jar until it was full and level to the top. "Is the jar full
now?" he asked. "No!" was the universal answer of the enlight-
ened class. "That is right," he responded. He proceeded to pour
sand over the gravel and big rocks. "Now, is it full?" he queried.
"No!" again the class rejoined.

He then lifted a container of water and filled the jar with
water right to the top of the rim. "Now is the jar full?" he asked
the class. "Yes!" They responded. "Okay, lets try a different
experiment," the teacher offered. He lifted a second large fragile
jar. He poured the same amount of water into the jar, then the

same amount of sand and an equal amount of gravel as he had placed in the first jar, but in reverse order. Then he tried to put in the same number of big rocks, but they would not fit. He asked the class, "What happened? Why can't I fit all the big rocks in?" "You need to put them in the jar in the right order," came the response. "That is right. So what are your big rocks in life? Have you placed them in your jar of life first? Do you have your priorities in order? Or, do you have sand and gravel that take up so much room you do not have time or energy for the big rocks?"

What are your big rocks in life? What are the things most important to you? If your home were burning up, what would you go for first? What is most vital to you-your telephone, the remote control, your CD collection, that novel you are reading, or your wardrobe? Or, would you get your children out of the house first? What are your highest priorities?

Plan Your Priorities

As a parent, do you live your life by planning your time, or as Stephen Covey teaches so well in his excellent book, *First Things First*, do you plan your priorities? At the beginning of each week, do you sit down and plan how you are going to meet your highest priorities? Is making sure you get to every piano, soccer and dance lesson the same level of importance as meeting your children's emotional needs? What are your highest priorities and how do you meet them? Think about this.

Which is more important-getting dinner on the table on time or listening to your child for just a minute? I know you may be thinking a minute is never enough. That is true if you do not start giving those minutes to your child until he is four years old. You have some make up work to do. You need to satisfy some unmet needs. But regardless of that, which is more important? Do you feed your child physically but not emotionally? If we fill their tummies with food but do not fill their hearts with tender love and honest caring, can the food ever give them all the nutrition they really need?

Change Your Life for the Better

By reading and practicing the steps found at the end of each section in this book, your entire perspective, and, in turn, your life, will change for the better. I guarantee it. Your children will enjoy better health than you ever imagined. They will blossom to display their grand potential. Your joy as a parent will expand to dimensions you have only briefly glimpsed in life.

Take a moment now and list your Big Rocks: List them in priority. Pick the top five in your life. At the end of your days, for what five things will you be the most grateful? Complete this exercise mindfully, because it will set the stage for the rest of the book.

1. _____
2. _____
3. _____
4. _____
5. _____

At least one of these values must be satisfied in every interaction with your children. Look over your list. Make sure no item is based on your kids' behavior or accomplishments. They should all reflect your own choices, growth and accomplishment.

Chapter 4
Do Your Children Ignore You?

There is nobody so irritating as somebody with less intelligence and more sense than we have.
—Don Herold

I want to share a powerful truth. Your children will stop paying attention to you when they have reached your age of emotional maturity. If your child is two years old and regularly tunes you out, maybe you need to grow up. This may sound harsh, but it is true. Give this idea careful consideration before you discard it. I saw a mother in a store looking at a product. She had a two-year-old child in the infant seat of her cart, and the cart was parked next to a display of appealing items. The child kept reaching for the tempting display. The mother repeatedly slapped her child's hand and would say, "Stop it," as she went back to reading labels. The mother never moved the cart, offered her child something better to do, or even paid any attention to the child, other than slapping the child's hand and barking out a command. The child would look at her mother and continue reaching for items on the shelves. The mother would ignore her for a moment and then repeat her command

and slap the child's hand again. The mother was behaving at the emotional level of a two-year-old. If she wanted the two-year-old to listen to her and honor her, she needed to grow up a little herself. If she had given the two-year-old something safe of equal appeal to entertain her, she could have been left to do her shopping, having directed her child's attention rather than choosing to be annoyed by her child's behavior.

Children Can Only Be Led

If your child at age thirteen is starting to tune you out, you need to go through a growth spurt of emotional and spiritual maturity. As parents, we must continue to grow and mature. As you practice the steps in this book with the insights and intentions outlined, you will grow emotionally, so you can lead your children to a higher level of maturity. Children can only be led. You can never chase a child to a higher awareness; you can only lead them.

Chapter 5
Discontent Is the Fertilizer for Growth

*A scholar who cherishes the love of comfort is not fit
to be deemed a scholar.*
—Lao-Tzu (570?- 490? BC)

If you have a level of discontent with your life as it is now, read on. You will find precious nuggets of truth, gems that add luster to life. Perfect health is a dream and a wish, but you can approach it by following the simple, but effective, activities taught in the following chapters. With stories, insights, and examples you can walk the invigorating path of discovery. Are you ready? Inspiration leads to perspiration, perspiration leads to realization, and realization leads to actualization. As you read, discover, and put to practice these simple steps, your experience in life will radically change and be better than ever before. Life Coach Tony Robbins said, "The very definition of insanity is to keep doing the same thing over and over again expecting a different result." Expect to change yourself in order to change your life experience.

Next you will learn the five essential aspects of health and the elements that create it. Fasten your seat belt; this is going to be exciting. . . .

Chapter 6
Saying I Love You, and Being Heard

If You Say I Love You, Do Your Children Hear?

"It doesn't matter how much I do for her, she never appreciates me."

"Tell me about her." I asked.

"She is so hard to get along with. She is always demanding more of me. I come home from work and have dinner to do, laundry, dishes from breakfast, the house to clean and she won't help or leave me alone. Being a single Mom is hard enough. She is so strong willed. If she doesn't get what she wants, she won't let anything else happen."

"Where do you think she learned that?"

"Oh definitely from me. Her dad is much easier going. But that's part of what makes me mad. He doesn't do anything for my daughter, and she still likes him more."

"Why do you think that?" I queried.

"It doesn't make any sense to me," she said with resignation.

Does this sound even a little familiar to you? Do you and your child not relate to one another? The answer to this draining situation is really not that hard. It is given to us each time we call one of our utility companies for service assistance anymore. The first question they ask is, "For help in English, press one. "Para ayudar en espanol, oprima el dos." We get to choose our language. In the easy to read and very helpful book *The Five Love Languages*, Gary Chapman teaches that there are five languages. Each of us wants to be shown in that language that we are loved. Just like we want to hear complex instructions in our native language, we want to be loved out of our native love language. If this lady's daughter only spoke Spanish and the mother was talking to her in English, the ability to communicate would have been less frustrating. But, unlike our native tongue, we have a very hard time learning a new love language.

So what is a love language?

Chapman defines five love languages. This is the way we want to be shown we are loved, meaning we feel affirmed, appreciated and accepted. The mother's love language in the above story was acts of service. The child's love language became apparent with just a question or two--it was words of affirmation. After talking about her daughter's love language, the mother went home, bent down to the daughter's height, looked her in the eye, and with great conviction told the daughter, "I want you to know that I love you and you are the most important thing in my life." Three days later the daughter was still on her best behavior and asked the mother several times, "Mom, am I still being good?" The mother was amazed at the power of one statement in the right language. The daughter heard the mother's statement in her heart, not only in her ears.

So what is your love language? What about your children? They will usually tell you if you listen. This little girl kept asking her mother, "Mom, do you love me?" The mother would say, "Of course, look at everything I do for you." The child would reply, "Perdoname, no entiendo loque' me dije'." Wrong language Mom. When she finally spoke in the daughter's language, the daughter responded beyond the mother's fondest desires. Was the one time speaking in the daughter's language enough? No, just a great beginning. So how do you find out what your love language is?

The five languages according to Chapman are:

- Words of Affirmation
- Acts of Service
- Receiving Gifts
- Quality Time
- Physical Touch

It is important to know your own love language so you can recognize when you are serving others out of it. It may be what you want, but it is possibly not the language they speak or understand. So how do you recognize the five love languages?

Physical touch is clearly spoken by children. If they show love by hugging, giving spontaneous kisses, rubbing your hand or arm or holding hands, then one of their love languages is physical touch. They need to be touched, held, cuddled and stroked. If not, they will not feel true acceptance, affection or appreciation, the three critical ingredients of feeling loved. You may be willing to sit all day, rubbing and stroking the child, but a child will receive any message more willingly if you are in gentle physical contact with them. To get their attention, touch them when speaking to them. When expressing appreciation, use the sign language of touch as well as the spoken word. Spend a moment every day with a child in your lap, if they need to be loved in this way.

Quality time is a breath of fresh air to the person who needs to be loved in this language. This child will love to go for a walk, just sit next to you on the couch, or have a story read to them. It doesn't much matter what activity is engaged in as long as you are with them. Giving your child your full attention is the gift of love they so crave to have instilled into their hearts.

Receiving gifts is not as hard a language to speak as you may fear. The gifts don't have to be extravagant or lavish. It is more the thought that counts than the size of the receipt. A single fresh flower is often as good as a dozen roses. A special note or a card is as valued as a more expensive doll. This child will often prize the gifts by storing them in a special place where they can be observed and cherished. They may hold on to these gifts too long in your opinion. Be careful not to diminish the importance of such old gifts. They symbolize the child's value in a way. Allow them to be retained if possible.

Acts of Service

Acts of service are given freely to children when they are young. Infants require constant care and nurture. As they age this need diminishes in some, but those who need acts of service still place great value on such simple acts. Help with homework, a special project, a broken bike, an item of clothing that needs mending are all acts of service that this child will hold dear. If your child constantly needs extra attention in some way like homework, maybe their love cup is feeling empty. So they get behind in homework so you need to let them know they are still loved. If you can give the gift freely, it has even more value. Watch carefully that you don't get behind in your deposits. You will see the signs once you recognize the language.

Words of affirmation or validation are a language that is easy to pick out. These children will often seek affirmation by asking for it. Do you like this mom? Did I do a good job? Do you like this? As a child, the affirming words came thick and fast. As children we all got lavished with words of affirmation, like "You are so cute or what beautiful eyes you have." Even homely children receive positive comments until around age three or four. Then those positive words get lost in the need for response from the parent or adult. These children, as most, will respond far more directly to positive words that honestly affirm their value and goodness.

For more information on this important topic please look up the book by Gary Chapman. It will make your life easier and much more satisfying in all your relationships.

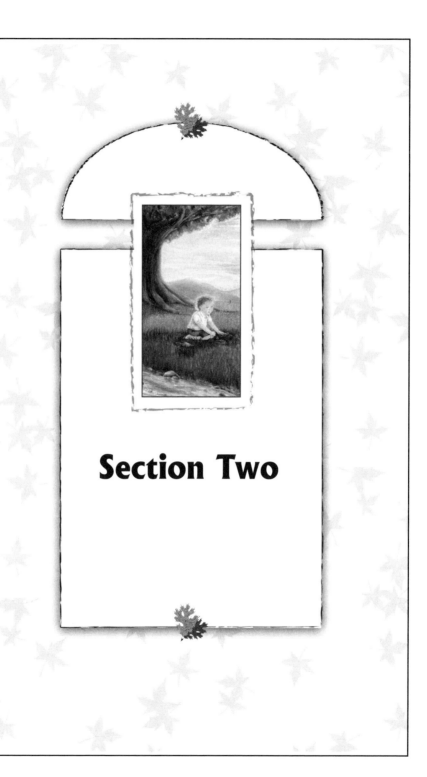

Section Two

Chapter 7
Gratitude: A Matter of Perspective

Men are not disturbed by things,
but the view they take of things.
—Epictetus (AD 55-135)

An ambulance speeds by with sirens wailing and lights flashing, shattering the calm of an early spring morning. What a disturbance, or is it? Each time an ambulance disrupts our peace, there is a deep shadow of distress resting on a family somewhere near. An event or a fright has possibly shaken their lives. A siren is not a disturbance; it is a call to gratitude. The shrill disruption is an opportunity to remember we have much for which to be grateful. This is a chance to expand our vision and to consider the wonders in our life we often take for granted. Once we see the good in our own lives, we can send our thoughts and prayers out to the home where the fresh shadow rests. Every flashing light is reminding us of the abundance we have and the challenges others are facing.

A Siren
Reading and pondering this book can be an ambulance siren, a call to awareness, and a call to gratitude. Our lives and

times are the most blessed in the history of the world. We have opportunities unrivaled. To take advantage of these expansive opportunities, we must be aware of the realities in which we live. We have opportunities never matched among any people for peace, prosperity, knowledge, and especially incredible health.

Pain: The Catalyst of Learning

A man's fortune must first be changed from within.
--Chinese Proverb

Good health gives us the chance to enjoy the extraordinary luxury of learning in the classroom of ease and abundance. In life, we usually need to have pain, trial, or challenge to be motivated to learn or change. Learning from trial and difficulty is much easier than learning in the midst of comfortable living. In life, learning from opposition is challenging. We seem to need the motivation of pain or discomfort to drive us from our current manner of thinking and being to a higher level of reality. Einstein reportedly stated, "No problem can be solved from the same level of consciousness that created it." Thus, to improve our state, at any level of life, we must change and improve our awareness. Learning in the midst of ease and prosperity comes from the pure inner soul's inspired desire for improvement. Learning under the stern, piercing eye of pain is easier but may leave us lacking in motivation and desire for the highest that is within us.

Increase Your Awareness

People seem to have a similar need for motivation with health. They are rarely grateful that the fourth toe on their left foot feels comfortable. No reflection is given to the patch of skin behind the right elbow that is soft and supple. We seem to take notice of our body only when health is lacking. With that lack of recognition comes a lack of motivation and incentive to stretch. We rarely improve our habits and traits while floating on the placid pool of ease and comfort. To enjoy true, vibrant health, increased awareness, effort, and focus are required.

Chapter 8
Building Health Destroys Disease

The death of dogma is the birth of reality.
—Immanuel Kant

This book is not intended to be a cure. The practices in this book are focused on health; a cure is focused on the disease. These steps at the end of each section are designed to build the positive attribute of health. Medication, surgery, and medical tests are all focused on disease, not on health. Every child, no matter what his or her problem, will be transformed by the application of these simple principles. This book is not intended to discourage you from seeing your children's medical practitioner but to make those services less necessary. As the level of health in your child or children grows and matures, you will not have to deal with illness. In the absence of illness and under the bright light of vibrant health, there is little needed input from your medical practitioner.

Be Proactive in Health
By following these simple steps, your family will learn proactive practices that will serve them in every life endeavor. To act proactively is to be prepared in all situations. Examples

of proactive health practices are ample sleep, good diet, regular exercise, emotional honesty, and spiritual awareness. To act proactively means you have the desired end in mind. To be proactive creates a desire for something that is good and gives birth to the characteristics needed to achieve that outcome.

Prevention is the act of moving away from the disease. The motive in moving away from disease is fear. Often in moving away from the sharp claws of one disease, we move directly into the open jaws of another. Proactivity in health is seeking a high level of wellness and acting in a way that will create that reality in your life. Proactivity requires being prepared by knowing your desired outcome and the way you need to be to achieve it. Preparation before the fact eliminates fear, which is the greatest single emotional state that results in disease. Fear is a precursor to illness. This will be discussed more fully in Section Three.

Chapter 9
The Building Blocks of Health

The way you think, the way you behave, the way you eat,
can influence your life by 30 to 50 years.
—Deepak Chopra

So what is health made of? There are five facets of health:

1. Spiritual
2. Emotional
3. Nutritional
4. Structural
5. Energetic

If you take the first letter in each category, you have the word SENSE. Vibrant health is made of the highest potential expressions in each level of the five facets of health. A balance in high qualities of SENSE, the five facets of health, constitutes optimum health. A balance in SENSE allows healing to occur in most situations. The body is a self-healing mechanism because God made it so. By using that ability at its highest level, we are manifesting the Creator's power within us. Our bodies were divinely created to heal. By fully accessing health, we are enhancing our divine potential.

"Your Body Is the Temple of God"

The construction of health is more than not feeling pain. It is more than the ability to press on regardless of your problems. To be ignorant of your body's needs, messages, lessons, and sensations is ignorance, not health. To be focused solely on our physical being is folly. We must find the "straight and narrow path" of balance during our walk in life. Once we find it and learn to navigate its narrow confines, we feel the liberation of a child who has just learned to ride a bike with no hands. Finding that path and learning to balance on it is not an easy task, but a vital life choice. Remember, as Paul so properly stated, "Your body is the temple of God." If we are to find the best within us, it is through our body, not despite it. Our spirit truly becomes the master of our soul by working with the body. This process of discovering the ability to tread the thin line of balance is health. To find out how to find and walk that thin line, continue to explore the depths of the following pages.

Chapter 10
Ask and Ye Shall. . .

*Beware when the great God lets loose a
thinker on this planet.*
—Ralph Waldo Emerson (1803-1882)

In the following pages, each section will provide an explanation of one category of SENSE. The end of each section will discuss simple strategies. When just one of the many suggestions is integrated, your child's potential to be healthy will improve. The more practices you integrate, the better the results. Are you satisfied reacting to ear infection after ear infection? Are you okay scrambling to accommodate the consistent demands of managing your children's illnesses? Stop being controlled by disease and start taking control of life and health by following the easy-to-apply strategies to improve your and your children's health.

The Laws of Health Are Simple

The laws of health are no different than the laws of nature. The Bible teaches, "Ask and ye shall receive, knock and it shall be opened unto you." It never says: "Pray that what you don't want to happen won't happen. Meditate on what you don't want to happen. Obsess on those things in life that are most frightening, and they will never occur. Worry about all that is negative, and it will never manifest in your life." Instead, it tells us to dream and plan what we want. If we ask and act congruently with that dream, we will find fascination in the dawning of our fondest imaginations.

Chapter 11
How Are You Motivated?

"Where there is no vision the people perish."
Bible

What is health? We talk about health and use it to describe a desirable state, yet we rarely define or study it. Almost all scientific studies are about disease. Why is this? People tend to be motivated by lack or absence, not abundance. They are often motivated by pain more than comfort. The United States became solidly unified after the attacks on September 11, 2001. This was because, in part, we lost our sense of security and had our fear brought to the forefront. The lack of security unified us as a whole. This is good, although not as good as if we are unified in an active pursuit of freedom for all, without the need for an attack on the safety of our society to encourage us.

Study Health

We are motivated to learn the most when we have a condition that frightens or challenges us. For this reason, most of our research money is spent to define and study disease. On the Internet, people in one month searched for information on breast health only 300 times, but searched for breast cancer 36,000 times. We seek to learn about disease when we have it. It may help us not be as sick, but understanding disease never helped anyone be truly healthy. Knowledge of disease may help you manage an illness or it may lend some comfort in an uncomfortable situation, but it will not help you be healthier.

How can we seek greater health if we do not study and define it?

Chapter 12
Health Is What?

You can free yourself from aging by reinterpreting your body and by grasping the link between belief and biology.
—Deepak Chopra

A good definition of health is the ability to comprehend yourself in your environment, spiritually, emotionally, nutritionally, structurally, and energetically.

When we comprehend ourselves in our environment, we understand ourselves and our environment at a deeper and more real level. We have a vivid awareness of our potential and possibility, and we are aware of the draw and pull of circumstances and our ability to stay centered in spite of them. With that comprehension comes the idea that the constant gravity-like pull to the highest and best that is in us--must come both from within and with inspiration from above. Given an opportunity, our body will heal itself. This opportunity begins with self-permission, which can only be given with an understanding of possibilities.

Enjoying optimum health means we have an understanding from each vantage point of SENSE:

Spiritual: Who we are, what our highest potential is, and how to achieve it helps define our spirituality. As we comprehend ourselves spiritually in our environment we begin to see ourselves as we really are in this stage of our existence, in context of our history and our possibility. It is out of this awareness that our thoughts, intents, desires, and actions originate. This awareness becomes the foundation for all growth and possibility in life.

Emotional: By comprehending ourselves in our environment emotionally, we understand why we are thinking what we think and why we feel what we feel. We will learn how to control our thoughts so we can act and not be acted on by the events in our life. If we understand ourselves clearly, we will recognize the true, inner power we have of unfettered choice. We come to see that every action, reaction, or lack of action comes from our own choice. Every situation brings us the possibility of liberation from something that holds us down and prevents us from full and free choice. To comprehend yourself in your environment is to see yourself clearly with the past, present, and future lain out before you. You enter a level of being that naturally engenders a high level of creativity. You can solve any problem to the advantage of all around you, because you have lost the need to support your unreal perceptions and beliefs. You will lose the need for a specific outcome. You are willing to see the wonder of the natural course in life. Soon you will prefer whatever occurs in your life. As the saying goes, "The Master prefers what occurs."

A great story is told of a teacher who was meditating with his students one day, while sitting by a small stream. During the mediation, the teacher heard a splashing sound in the stream. Looking down, he saw that a scorpion had fallen into the water. Scorpions do not swim well. Without hesitation, he reached down and lifted the scorpion out of the water and set it on the bank. As soon as the scorpion touched the ground, it stung the teacher in the hand. He calmly went back to meditating. In a few minutes, the splashing sound came again from the stream. Again, the scorpion had fallen into the water. The teacher reached down again without hesitation to save the scorpion from drowning. One of his students interrupted him and said, "Master, if you pick up the scorpion, he will sting you again. Why would you do that?" The teacher said, "It is the nature of the scorpion to sting, this I know. But it is my nature to save. I will not let his nature control my nature." He picked up the scorpion and put it on the bank.

When we find our true nature we have the ability and power to choose for ourselves our actions in all circumstances and situations. When we develop the power to act, we no longer need to react.

Nutrition: Our body exists to teach us. It is not to be our master but our tutor. If we are cautious and aware, we can learn to hear its messages. Nutrition is one way for us to blend our physical, spiritual, and emotional being with nature. By eating properly, we harmonize with our environment. As we eat properly, as described in Section 6, we blend our internal physiology with nature and stay balanced despite the pull of climate, season, and weather. We are then able to stay centered with our environment.

Structure: Our structure, meaning the physical tissues of the body, is a vivid external manifestation of our inner reality. The way we carry ourselves, the posture we hold, and the care we give our protective frame are reflective of our inner integrity. Our structure protects our grand communication system, the nerve system. The integrity of our nerve system is critical to self-awareness. Self-awareness and balance in our structural system are essential to maintaining and improving health. Abraham Lincoln is credited with saying: "Your parents are responsible for your face until age forty. You are responsible for the appearance of your face after."

Energy: All matter is made of energy. There are many methods that teach awareness on an energetic level. Learn about our energetic nature and how to create energetic balance in section 8. It is crucial to dynamic health.

Chapter 13
Your Body Is a Self-healing Machine

The greatest mistake you can make in life is to be
continually fearing you will make one.
—Unknown

When we create the ability to perceive ourselves in our environment, the body's natural inclination to heal will take place at a highly efficient rate. The human body is a self-healing mechanism. A cut on your finger will heal with little attention on your part. The same is true thousands of times a day throughout your body. Our ability to perceive ourselves in our environment is the capacity to recognize our environment and correctly choose the most efficient and effective path to full and vibrant health within the realities of that environment. If we are unable to achieve our full potential because we misread our situation, we will simply adapt to the best of our ability. This adaptation is a common cause of many chronic health problems. We settle for adaptation instead of healing. If our recognition of the outside environment or our inner healing mechanism is not correct, our response will be less than appropriate. The result will be an imbalanced adaptation and less than optimal health.

This is exemplified by conditions like allergies, which are an abnormal reaction to a normal environmental substance. Some people react to dust by sneezing, having a stuffy nose, puffy eyes, and other symptoms of allergies. Other people can breathe in the same dust and have no response at all. The problem is not in the dust, but our response to a normal, environmental substance. By helping the body perceive itself and the environment more clearly, the need to react abnormally is resolved. I have personally experienced hundreds of cases of allergies relieved naturally by use of an approach called NAET, Nambudripad's Allergy Elimination Technique. Autoimmune disorders such as multiple sclerosis, lupus, and Crohn's disease all are incorrect responses within the body to common stressors. The body believes it needs to attack itself to adapt to its environment, when the body's reaction is, indeed, the major cause of the condition and the symptoms that follow. As the body truly comprehends itself in its environment or understands its physiological needs and the real impact of the environment, it will not attack normal tissue in an effort to stay balanced. It will seek to heal and restore these tissues in a continuing cycle of restoration that is normal to our nature. These are only a few of the myriad situations of the body not comprehending itself in its environment. Therefore, we may be able to diagnose and manage a disease, but if we restore health fully, the disease will have no root to grow and will disappear.

When we see the real, underlying cause, we can choose to eliminate it from our being. True health is a noteworthy objective in life, if our desire is to live up to our highest potential.

Chapter 14
Nature's Balance

Baseball is ninety percent mental and
the other half is physical.
—Yogi Berra

Every characteristic of nature has an opposite balancing character such as hot and cold, day and night, desert and rain forest, heaven and earth, male and female, masculine and feminine. Health is made up of a balance of these dualities. When our system is balanced in this simple but profound system, we are naturally healthy. When our immune function is neither too active nor too passive, we are in balance or in health. If our circulation is neither too much nor too little, we are in balance and, thus, in health. This balance can only come if we comprehend ourselves in our environment.

One duality, light and dark, is fascinating. We can describe light as an oscillating electromagnetic wave or particle within our visible range of perception. Darkness defies solitary definition; it is just the lack of light. It has no mass, shape, size, texture, color or energy. It is a lack of light--it is really nothing. But, because we understand light, we also understand the antithesis of light—darkness.

Imagine going into a deep cave with flashlights as our guide. After walking on the cool, wet, rocky path for thirty minutes, we are deep in the earth. We turn off our flashlights. The chill of the absolute darkness surrounds us. It rests on us like a heavy, wet blanket. You are given a broom and asked to use it to sweep the darkness away to be able to see again. Could you do it? How about if you were given a shovel or even a snowplow? It cannot be done unless you introduce light. By bringing light into the cave, darkness will flee.

The same rules apply to health and disease. Health is like light, and disease is like darkness. A disease, like darkness, can only exist when there is no health or light. If a room is fully lit, darkness cannot exist, unless there is some object that blocks the light. If the room is completely bathed in light, darkness cannot be present. A human body that is fully healthy cannot harbor disease. If a person's pancreas is perfectly healthy, diabetes cannot exist. If the coronary arteries and heart tissue and circulation are fully healthy, a heart attack is not possible.

Disease Is Lack of Health

By all accounts disease is just a lack of health. If health in all its characteristics and attributes is present, disease cannot exist. So the entity that we study so vigorously, disease, is in reality, a nonentity. It is only a lack of its tangible counterpart: health. As darkness cannot be pushed out of a room without introducing light, disease cannot ever be pushed out of a body without introducing a higher degree of health.

Chapter 15
Wisdom from the Child

*There is nobody so irritating as somebody with less
intelligence and more sense than we have.*
—Don Herold

When my youngest daughter, Jenna, was in the first grade,
we attended a parent teacher conference. Her teacher told the
following story. One day she gave an assignment to the class to
think of something they were good at and write about it. The
kids each picked a topic and began the task. The next day the
teacher asked the kids to write about something they could not
do and were not good at and why they were not good at it. All
the kids bent over their desks, picked up their pencils, and
started writing. The teacher said Jenna sat for a minute looking at her paper and then spent the rest of the time looking
around the class. This was very unlike Jenna. She always got
right to her work and was one of the first children finished with
her assignments. She never even picked up her pencil. When
the teacher informed the students time was about almost up,
Jenna quickly picked up her pencil and wrote a short sentence.
The teacher said she was fascinated. In more than twenty years

of teaching, she had never had a child respond as Jenna had for this assignment. The papers were handed in and the children excused to recess. The teacher quickly shuffled through the papers to see what Jenna had written. She found her paper and, with interest, read her response. In a short sentence, she answered the question "What are you not good at?" in a simple and profoundly correct way. She had written, "I just do my best, and that's good enough."

That is what I hope each of you will do. That is all you and your children ever need to do-your best. "And that's good enough."

Chapter 16
Creating Health

Pick battles big enough to matter, small enough to win
—Jonathan Kozel

We must look at the idea of creating health from a positive place of desire and passion. We must seek a healthier lifestyle by positive intention with a firm grasp on the desired outcome. If the objective is to live life with the goal of vibrant health, we will most likely achieve that outcome. If we live life hoping to avoid disease, at best we will delay the inevitability of creating that which we focus on--disease. We will never achieve a truly healthy existence and will inhibit the full enjoyment of our daily lives, as well as our ability to express our full potential. We will be limited and will neither experience the abundant joy this life has to offer nor share with others the full measure of our truest nature.

Would you like to find the secrets to creating powerful self-esteem for your child? Would you like your child always to know who he or she really is and act out of his or her own choices instead of bowing to peer pressure? Discovering your spiritual potential and, in turn, leading your children to recognize theirs is the key. In each of the following sections, I will share simple steps essential to activate your children's spiritual appetite, emotional balance, nutritional harmony, physical integrity, energetic awareness, and dramatically increase your ability to create these realities in your home. These simple, daily activities cannot fail to brighten the life of every member of your family when followed.

For twenty years, I have explored the mountains and valleys of health. How do we acquire it? How do we maintain it? How do we define it? Read the next five sections, and you will begin to glimpse the vast possibilities that lay before you. Read them again, and your understanding will deepen. Each time you apply one principle, the others will take on a different light. I encourage you to read the book over and over again. If you want to see your child in a more positive light than ever before, to have your parenting batteries recharged, to make life fresh and fun again, then read on. Prepare for the light inside to be turned on and see your children for what they are: Children of Promise. Read on and discover the extent of the promise.

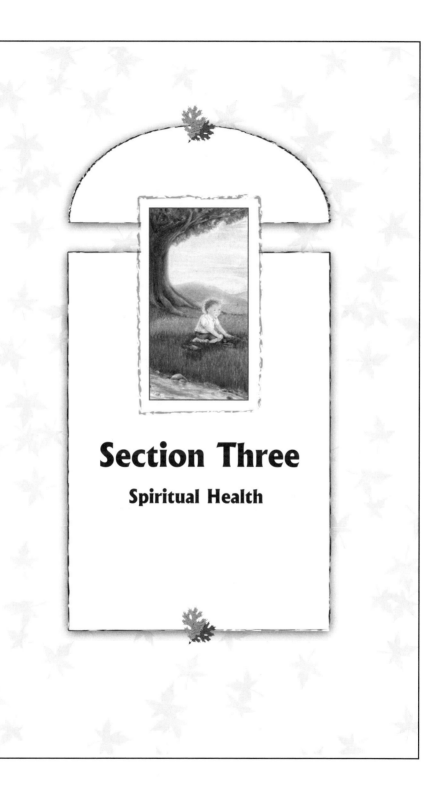

Section Three

Spiritual Health

Chapter 17
The One Source of Wisdom

I want to know God's thoughts...the rest are details.
—Albert Einstein

Much is written and practiced on the topic of spirituality. It seems people practice the system, usually as contained in a religion they were exposed to when they were young, or else they flee as far as possible from what they were presented with during their youth. Both paths create inherent challenges. In the first scenario, people tend to practice without personal consideration what they were taught as a youth. It may be difficult to mature in that system, because it is rarely scrutinized, challenged, or evaluated, and thus not strengthened or even understood. The flaws and fears of previous generations can be carried down through the years without reconsideration of their value or purpose.

In the second case, people deny all that was given to them and flee to the farthest philosophical island they can find. As is the case in most situations, the best practice lies between the two extremes; it is a balance. Balance is a vague term, but it holds a powerful meaning, and it is a topic that will come up over and over again as we seek to discover SENSE.

Seek the Verifiable Path

At the very least, the path of spirituality we choose should be proved and qualified individually. The ability to gain a spiritual certainty that we are on a true path for the attainment of our highest potential must be substantiated. There must be a way to validate the path in our heart, as well as in our mind. They both must speak peace to our soul. Seek the verifiable path. In the Bible the book of James, chapter one, verse five says "If any of you lack wisdom let him ask of God. . .and it shall be given him." Ask, and we will receive. Ask, and it will take us on a winding path of the explorer of truth. It will require determination, gratitude, and especially humility, but as we journey down this pathway, our spirituality will be deepened, our passion for life enlivened, and our joy will be expanded.

Chapter 18
The Still and Small Voice

A man should look for what is, and not for
what he thinks should be.
—Albert Einstein

The truly spiritual binds us to the divine. There are many influences to which we can subject ourselves and become aware. Most have the capacity to expand our view in some way. To keep it simple, that which has the capacity to draw us to God, or if you prefer the divine, will be referred to as "spiritual." That which is spiritual causes the divine to infiltrate every aspect of our lives. Gifts of awareness and intuition should not be confused with spiritual aspects of our nature. These gifts have a different function. The spiritual aspect of our nature is deep and quiet within us. The divine voice is still and small. We must be attentive and aware of our deepest senses to attune to this still and quiet voice within us. The spiritual part within us is much more like a slow and deep running river than a thundering rapid or babbling brook. It makes little sound but has a deep and powerful current.

Chapter 19
The Foundation of Spirituality

"The fool hath said in his heart, There is no God."
Psalm 14:1

Of what is spirituality made? First, spirituality requires the recognition of who we and who our children really are. By all accounts, we are the product, creation, and most accurately, the offspring of God. As such, we have a specific and incredible divine potential and an awesome heritage. We are children of God—not just the creations of, but children of, God. We are, as has been well-stated, spiritual beings having a mortal experience rather than mortal beings seeking a spiritual experience. We are not just spiritual beings, but also spirit beings. That which drives our mind is our spirit self. When we die, because we are spirit beings, we will maintain our individuality. Our physical body will die, but we continue to live, even though our body will be left a cold shell once we pass on. It is as a horse to a cowboy. If the horse dies, the cowboy still continues. Our spirit, the real and permanent "us" is made of matter more fine and pure than our current ability to discern. Nonetheless, it is very real and authentic.

51

Numerous accounts are recorded of people who have experienced out of the body events where they left their physical body, traveled around, saw and heard verifiable conversations and activities in areas distant to their body, then returned to wake and recount the experience to a nearby nurse or visitor. These experiences relating remote activities proved to be precisely true. One of the amazing things is that they could use their senses when out of the body and then recall the memories on returning. It must be our sprit, not our body, that composes our mind.

Chapter 20
Spirituality Impacts Health

I am ready to meet my Maker. Whether my Maker is prepared for the great ordeal of meeting me is another matter.
—Sir Winston Churchill (1874-1965)

`How does spirituality impact health? How is it part of health? How do we exercise and increase our spirituality and that of our children? How do we recognize, in all situations, our children's divine heritage and treat them accordingly? This section will give simple steps that will strengthen our spirit self and that of our children. These steps will help to integrate into our children the powerful recognition that they are children of God; therefore, they are inherently good and wonderful. They will look at themselves in the mirror and see the reflection of the divine. Self-judgment, condemnation, criticism, and dislike will be dismantled. Self-esteem, self-appreciation, recognition of true talents and abilities, self-forgiveness, and honest love for self will be given a fertile soil in which to grow. The Bible teaches that we are to love our neighbor as ourselves. Self-love is the beginning of love for our neighbor and love of God. By loving yourself, you are then open to receive the love of others. Until we love ourselves, the love of God and the love from others are difficult to receive. As we are willing to experience the beginning of self love, we open ourselves to receive God's love, as well as the love of others. As we begin to feel the love of God in our lives, the tendency to seek and do the will of God grows. By seeking and doing the will of God, our ability to feel God's love matures, and we become more godly creatures. When we seek the will of God because it is our desire and nature, we begin to change into our potential and to fulfill our promise. Righteous self-love, which is really the only type of self-love, precipitates consciously accepting the love of God and giving your love to God and your fellowmen. We cannot practice unrighteous self-love; it is really not love at all but pride and egotism. Self-love can only be righteous love or right love or godly love.

A young girl was asked by her teacher, "If you could spend the day with anyone, who would it be?" Her response was, "I would spend the day with myself because I like myself, and there isn't anything wrong with that." This attitude is both refreshing and delightful. Many of us do not know what to do with ourselves on a rainy Saturday afternoon. What a blessing to find your own company enjoyable, exciting, and invigorating!

Chapter 21
Please, Tell Me What You Mean

I have found the best way to give advice to your children is to find out what they want and then advise them to do it.
—Harry S Truman (1884-1972)

The following story teaches a vital point of awareness for all parents. A young father was at the airport awaiting the arrival of family members on an incoming flight. He had his young son with him. As they sat waiting, the son, becoming more comfortable with the surrounding environment, started playing and wandering farther and farther from his father. At one point, the little boy wandered around a nearby corner just out of the view of his father. The father got up quickly and picked his boy up and said, "Do not go around the corner." The boy looked up at him in a defiant manner and promptly walked around the corner again. The young father, worried for his child's safety, got up again and brought the son back and said, "Do not go around the corner." The boy looked at the father again and in brash defiance walked around the corner again. The father feeling the need to emphasize the lesson, stood up, picked him up again, and this time lightly spanked him. Sternly, he scolded the child, "Do not go around the corner." The child with tears in his eyes looked up at his father and again promptly walked around the corner. "Okay, if this is the way you want it," the father replied. He got up, stalked around the corner and this time swatted the child's fanny with a few good, firm swats. Then, setting him down, he said one more time, "Do not go around the corner." With tears in his eyes, the child looked up at the father and asked, "What's a corner?"

Chapter 22
Every Child Is Unique and Extraordinary

There are powers inside of you, which, if you could discover and use, would make of you everything you ever dreamed or imagined you could become.
—Orison Swett Marden

Wise parents always make sure that they are so clear about their expectations for their children, and of their motives for those expectations, that those expectations can never be misunderstood.

It is vital to recognize that our children may have talents and personalities that are different from our own. A child like us may be easier to understand, communicate with, and can be comforting to a parent. It is the child who seems to come from another planet that makes us pause and think and provides an opportunity to grow outside our current self-imposed limits. That child simply sees life differently. There was a school class where the children were drawing pictures. The teacher asked one young girl what she was drawing. The girl proudly said, "I am drawing a picture of God."

"Well, we do not know what God looks like," the teacher responded.

"Wait until I am done and then you will know," replied the girl.

Please be patient and recognize that it is our job as parents to understand where they are coming from, not to make them conform to your way of looking at the world. Our job is to find and help them cultivate all the goodness that dwells in them. Activities will be given at the end of the section to provide extra tools for deeper understanding. Just remember that all children come into this world good. These tools will assist in helping you find the fullness of a child's natural goodness.

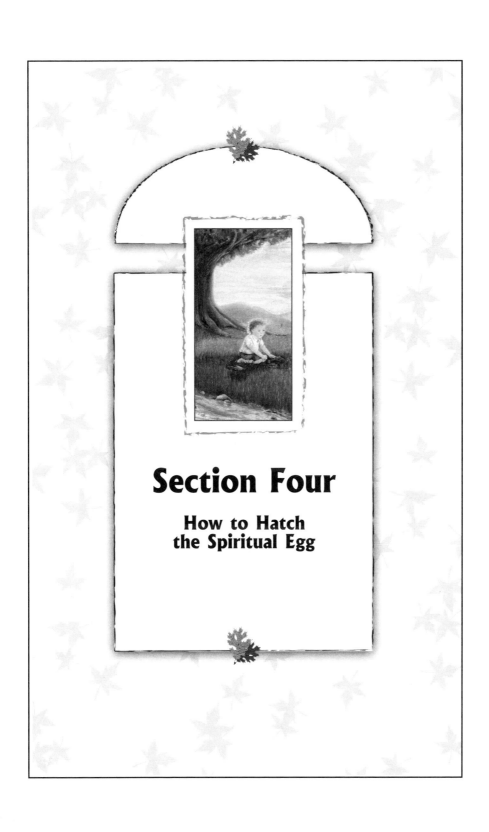

Section Four

How to Hatch
the Spiritual Egg

Chapter 23
Activities for Bringing the Spirit to the Surface

There is always one moment in childhood when the door opens and lets the future in.
—Deepak Chopra

Prayer

Prayer is the intentional effort to commune with divinity on divinity's terms. We do not get to set the terms of our interaction on a spiritual level and receive a deep spiritual experience.

Prayer is where we find the way to interact with God for our benefit and the benefit of others. As we do this, we develop gratitude, honesty, inner knowingness, and a desire for self-improvement.

Prayer can and should be instinctive. We can use memorized or scripted prayers. A full prayer experience opening our heart in honest expression of our deepest feelings will result in a tighter bond with God. Converse with God like you do with your most trusted friend and confidant.

Prayer becomes most effective when we are willing to submit our will to God's will. God will then usually grant us that which we desire. When we are willing and happy to do whatever God wants, even if it is hard, then we can receive what we want from God, because it will be one in the same.

Prayer is also effective when we are absolutely willing to do whatever it is God puts into our heart. When we are willing to do God's will, we will usually understand what it is. Then we must act.

Few attributes are more powerful than a prayerful heart. As a parent, we gain greater power through prayer than any other medium. We will not gain power over our children but over ourselves. When we learn to draw on the powers of heaven, our children will learn to draw on us.

Meditation

Meditation is a dynamic and soulful practice. It quiets our inner voices and centers us on our true nature. Creativity is unleashed in meditation. By practicing and teaching our children meditation, we teach them that they do not have to be busy to be of value. It also teaches the value of self-responsibility. It will help you, as the parent, and your child increase in creativity. Greater self-awareness grows with the fertilization of meditation. Sit in a comfortable chair with your feet flat on the floor, palms in your lap, eyes closed but looking just slightly upward; be quiet and mindful. Listen to your thoughts, ideas, and desires. Ponder on possibilities and solutions to life's opportunities. Answers will come; ideas will flood your mind and heart. Get in touch with yourself; you may also find you like being with you.

Contemplation

Encourage your children to take time to contemplate their situations in life. Ask them what they think about their situation and their options. Help them see the limitless options they have. Thomas Edison once said, "When you have exhausted all the possibilities, remember this, you haven't." Encourage them to ponder on even simple dilemmas until they understand how to do it on their own. Help them see each situation in unique and different ways. One of the great dangers in life is to lose the ability to be creative in our perception. To do things in life just because that is the way we have seen it done or have done it is a great obstacle to growth and potential. Contemplation is not worrying. Contemplation is focusing on the positive possibilities that always exist in life. Look at life with the willingness to learn from every situation. Teach your children the same ability.

Choose the most desirable options to act on. Always be creative in solving dilemmas. If we are creative, so will our children be creative. Once in a junior high school, where the girls exerted their creativity, they put their lipstick on and then kissed the mirror, leaving lip prints on the glass. The principal and janitor jointly devised a solution. They invited the girls they believed were the culprits to the restrooms and quickly explained how this habit created extra work for the janitor. In fact, the principal asked the janitor to show the girls just how difficult it was to get the lipstick off the mirrors. The janitor moved to the front of the group, and with a little flourish, he stepped to a toilet, dipped the squeegee into the bowl, and wiped the mirror down with it. The girls were aghast. The mirrors they were kissing had been cleaned with toilet water. Yuck! The problem ended that day. Be creative in problem solving. Think out of your box.

A Moment of Quiet Time or Prayer

Prayer and/or meditation morning and evening provides opportunity to assess the day before it begins and evaluate it after it has passed. It gives us another chance to be fully present. These will draw your family closer to God as you approach God in humble prayer. Prayer is an opportunity to thank more than to ask and a very important time to talk to God and, especially, to listen as quiet, warm impressions fill your heart. If you choose meditation, you can ask the family for as much time as they are capable of giving quietness. At different ages it will vary. Different children will have different abilities. Give them an easy way to end their session. When they are finished meditating, they can get up and gently touch each member of the family on the cheek as they go to their rooms. When all of the children are done, you can go tuck them into bed.

A Prayer of Gratitude at Each and Every Meal

Expression of gratitude for the abundant blessings we have received is an opportunity, as well as an obligation. Nutrition is one of our major avenues of connecting ourselves with our environment in healthy living. Doing so mindfully is both wise and necessary for a balanced physical/spiritual nature. Teach your children to put down their fork or spoon between each bite. Chew the food well. Be aware of the chewing process. It is the first step to digestion. Good digestion protects us from a myriad of undesirable conditions.

Special Prayers, Contemplation, or Meditation for Special Events

Any special circumstance, need, or event is appropriate to seek a special spiritual connection and guidance. Any sincere approach to God in prayer will draw you and your child closer to seeing things as God does or as they really are. This will help in daily choices, as well as choices in unusually challenging events.

Teach Children the Principle of "Ask and Ye Shall Receive"

In the Bible, Christ taught repeatedly the truth of "ask and ye shall receive." This law is irrevocably tied to the law of the harvest. "As you sow so shall you reap." The innermost desire in your heart, when you prayerfully ask, will determine the response to your petition. If our inner desire is selfish in any way, we will get an answer, not the one we want but the one we need. Through consistent prayer we come to learn of our true inner desires. We begin to be able to ask with awareness exactly for that which we would like to have. As we become more and more aligned with the will of God, we ask for that which God already has in store for us and would have us receive. And as we ask in that way, our desires come into union with God's desires for us, and it "shall be given unto you."

Chapter 24
Taste the Good Word of God

The task of the modern educator is not to cut down jungles,
but to irrigate deserts.
—*C. S. Lewis*

Study Spiritual Literature Daily

Spend some time, even as little as two minutes, reading some deeply spiritual literature every day. This can be done at the beginning or end of the day. If the children are young, it will invite an attitude into the home that will be vividly felt by these very sensitive little ones. This atmosphere will cultivate a deeper yearning and craving for things that carry the feel of the spiritual. If you, as a parent, demonstrate a deep love for spiritual literature, your children will form an appetite for it also.

They may not remember the words, but they will remember how they felt in that experience. It will also draw us and our children closer to the divine and to the accompanying characteristics of kindness, gentleness, gratitude, meekness, love, and a deep inner self-confidence that can only come from a stronger connection with God. Make this activity a "get to" instead of a "have to." Make sure the session includes personal touch, closeness, and a good feeling. Do not force children to be perfect. Just let them know their presence is the most important thing. Always finish with a hug. A hug is something children always enjoy, and be creative with your hugs. They do not always have to be regular hugs. We used to use a bear hug, a monkey hug, or a squirrel hug. The kids got to imagine what a monkey hug was like, and we would hug the way they thought monkeys would hug. Be creative, and the time together will be more rewarding. Make sure the kids are the center of the process, and they will love it even more.

Share Your Feelings about Things of a Spiritual Nature

Do not hesitate to be a little emotional if you feel it. I still remember my mother emotionally sharing her conviction of God and her relationship with God. Even though I had no interest in those things at that time of my life, I knew they were real and important to her. As I matured, I knew that I wanted to find the peace my mother had, so I sought out my own path with her example as my guiding light. Never hesitate as a parent to use this time to extend an appropriate apology for the mistakes that we as parents frequently make.

Always take the appropriate moment to express your love to your children and tell them how much they mean to you as individuals. There are appropriate moments every day. They need to know it and believe it.

Chapter 25
Time, the Gift of Love

Yesterday is ashes, tomorrow wood.
Only today does the fire burn brightly.
—Eskimo Proverb

Family Time

- Plan a weekly family event. A specific night of the week is best. Make it a "Big Rock." Make sure it always happens. This will bring blessings in your home that no other activity can.

- The core of this event should occasionally be of a spiritual tone. Begin with a prayer, a small reading of a spiritual nature, a song, or a moment of meditation.

- It also needs to be fun and enjoyable. This is often a challenge. Start with planning the fun and then work in a spiritual lesson.

- Uplifting music can be a positive, contributing factor.

- Sharing positive stories about your youth is very mean - ingful. Be careful not to tell the same stories over and over again. And do not start with: "When I was young..." They will soon tune you out.

- Some type of treat in the form of food or a game is a good way to end the event.

- End with a prayer or moment of silent meditation expressing gratitude for each member of your family and the chance to be together. Find the positive to pray about or express to each family member.

Chapter 26
Unclutter Your Thoughts

I have found the best way to give advice to your children is to find out what they want and then advise them to do it.
—Harry S. Truman

Journal writing is a wonderful pathway to self-awareness. Writing and drawing in a journal is a great way to express deep, inner feelings. This helps children find ways to understand their spiritual and emotional feelings. This activity can be part of your "family time." Drawing and scrap booking will give you great insight into the child's view of common family events. I remember a picture drawn by my oldest daughter when she was very young. It had stick figures of my two daughters and my wife with the typical body, legs, and arms with the circle head on top. I was standing next to them, but I was drawn with no body, just very long legs, and a head, and two arms sticking out of the legs. I was puzzled for a moment as to why I was drawn so differently. Then I realized to her, being as small as she was, I looked like that, being 6´3´´. I was just a long set of legs with a head on top. It was then I realized I didn't get down on the ground at my children's level nearly enough.

Journal writing has also been shown to improve immune function. Improved immune function will protect children from the myriad of colds, flu's, and other "bugs" that are so pervasive in our society. Children can be encouraged to write on a myriad of topics.

A daily gratitude journal is also tremendous. Write about what they like in other people. They can write about their favorite friends, pets, imaginary friends, and activities. They could write about what they would like to do on their next vacation. They could describe what their ideal day would be like. They can be encouraged to tell about their favorite oocurence each day, what they would like to do over again if they could, what words they wish they hadn't said, or what they would like to say to someone but didn't dare to say.

Select Television Viewing Wisely

Provide alternative and often better activities for children. One mother asked a grown son when he first learned to love to read. Even though she had made it a consistent effort to read to him from his youth, he said, "It was when you blew up the TV." From the ages of eight to fourteen, children form huge numbers of neuronal pathways. These are brain pathways that give us the ability to learn, perform, and participate at a high level in a wide variety of activities. Children preserve only those neuron or brain pathways they use repetitively. Plan and encourage various forms of activities for your children that use all their senses.

Writing helps to develop their vocabulary. Challenge them to come up with different words to describe a commonly used term. "Creatively challenged" can be used to describe stupid or dumb. Even though not the best term, it is a step in the right direction to seeing things in a more real way and to frame them in a positive light.

The more activities and games children participate in that challenge the various senses and thinking skills, the better the new neuronal pathways will be retained. Encourage an active mind. Get your children to tell you stories that they make up. Make up bedtime stories for them.

I know one man who paid his children allowances based on

the books they read and reported on. He provided the list of acceptable books. As the children read those mind-expanding books and wrote a report describing what they had learned from that book, he paid them a fair allowance.

Encourage your children to create with their hands. Drawing, making clay figures, beading, and playing with small hand toys all encourage manual dexterity and preservation of potential talents and skills. As adults, we would be wise to participate with our children in these activities also. You never know what a child's latent talents might be until he gets a chance to express them. Honest self-expression through creativity is one way to connect with the most sacred parts of your soul. That which you create models your assumed nature. This is another good reason to avoid many of Hollywood's ragged expressions of creativity.

Chapter 27
The Quality of Your Questions Matter

Any intelligent fool can make things bigger and more complex.... It takes a touch of genius- and a lot of courage to move in the opposite direction.
—Albert Einstein

Help your children learn that they are a spirit being first and foremost. Questions are the key to this level of growth. Always help them ask better questions. Find out why they ask the questions they ask. What is it they really want to understand? Help them create a better question and then find the answers. Art Linkletter made a career out of children's questions and innocent answers to questions. What we sometimes see as annoying, incessant questions from a child may be a plea for recognition. Maybe they do not need an answer as much as attention. Your attention can never be used in a better way than the formation of a human being. No casserole, dirty room, laundry, business project, or TV show is as important as your children. Try and remember that and honor their real needs. There is an answer to every question. A parent's greatest challenge is to understand the real question.

71

Our youngest daughter at a surprisingly young age asked my wife a great question. As they were in the car one day, she took advantage of a stoplight to ask my wife, "Hey Mom?"

"Yes?" my wife distractedly responded.

"I have just one question." This has always been a warning shot over the bow from this daughter. "Why can you pick my nose and I can't?"

What was she really asking here? Was it really about picking her nose? No. She was wondering why adults and kids have different privileges. It was a great question and one that deserved an honest discussion.

Parenting Is Not a Contest

Find out what your child is really trying to ask. Ask them about their questions. Do you want to know...? Is what you are asking. . . ? What do you think the answer to that question might be? Answer the question and then ask them what they think about your answer. Ask them how they feel about the answer. Ask them to give their answer to the question. Always honor their questions with a compliment and an honest response. Help them develop the ability to ask good, deep questions.

One young boy asked his father, "Dad, what color is a mirror?" Realize that some children are very different in nature, gifts, personality, and disposition than their parents. Some questions will seem perhaps silly and sometimes just plain senseless to you. There are no silly questions, because questions always come from deep within our being. Most questions arise from a desire to find one's self. Seek to understand the child and the miracle he or she is. Try never to show the child you are better, smarter, or superior to them.

Parenting is not a contest to see who is most powerful. You may be smarter or stronger, but proving that is not a recipe for helping your child develop the confidence to honor who he is at his best. Children are our challenge and our gift. They challenge our ability to express our understanding and views of life, love, and the universe. They are our gift by keeping us humble, centered, and stretching each and every day. Children give us the chance to develop the virtue of love by being the easiest and most lovable creatures on the face of the earth. They provide us the privilege to enter on the pathway of love. If we cannot love our children, loving ourselves is probably beyond our ability. As we love them, we grow in ways never before possible. As we learn to love them, we can begin to love ourselves. We not only see our children as incredible, but we see life as incredible and ourselves as a deserving partner in the wonder of life.

The promise of this book is that as the children heal, so do the parents; as parents grow, so do the children. As the children learn to love, so do the parents. As the children learn to look at the wonders of life and say, "Wow!" so do the parents.

Chapter 28
A Loan From God

What a man thinks of himself, that is what determines, or
rather indicates, his fate.
—Henry David Thoreau

Remember who your children are. They are not your possessions; they are just on loan from God. We do not own them, but we do have an obligation to love them, honor them, learn from them, help them understand themselves as they really are, and to help them see their true, highest potential. Christ taught a simple deep truth when he said: "Suffer the little children to come unto me, for of such is the kingdom of heaven." As we let them keep the wonders that make them heavenly and grow into sweet maturity, we will all be able to "stand all amazed" at the wonder of this mortal existence, of this incredible plan of happiness we are a part of every day. The fact that God trusted you with them is a sign you are up to the task. You can be a great parent. You are the right person to be caring for that bundle of spirit, energy, and love. I believe they accepted you as parent, and you accepted them as your children before you came here. God proclaimed you up to the task when they came into your life. Take confidence in that fact. Be confident in your ability to honor that task. You may not be perfect, but you are called to do a job you are up to.

Service and Kindness Counteract Depression

Commend your child for his or her kind and unselfish acts. Ask how it felt to perform this act of kindness. When we do something nice for another person, our brain chemistry shifts, and our serotonin levels rise. Serotonin is one of the chemicals that counteract the state of depression. Service and kindness counteract depression. Seeing a kind act, doing an act of kindness, or receiving an act of kindness will all regulate our molecules of emotion and help us feel our best.

As we serve our children, they see first hand an example of a Christ-like characteristic. They learn to reach outside of themselves and to be difference makers in the world. They will learn to give of themselves in a healthy way. This is really the only way to get anything meaningful in life; give of your inner-self from the gifts God has placed in you. Share your gifts out of a pure motive, and all will benefit.

Chapter 29
Purpose in Life

Man is that he might have joy.
—Joseph Smith

Last, help them work toward finding their purpose in life. This is the discovery and vivid awareness of their highest potential, even as it applies beyond this mortal life. Why are we on this mortal journey? What is our highest potential? Help your children gain a working knowledge and understanding of this foundational principle of spiritual awareness and actuality. It just might stretch you a little. Our purpose should not fall only within the boundary lines of mortality. A noble purpose can and should extend beyond this life to the next phase of our existence. I will discuss this in terms of your purpose. It will be difficult to help your children think about their purpose if you have not first pondered and discovered the beginnings of your own.

Purpose

One day, we will all give an accounting for our mortal life. On stating our accomplished life purpose, if it is honorable and we have lived it, we will receive a rejoining, "Well done thou good and faithful servant." Let your purpose and that of your children extend beyond the mortal phase of our existence. I know one dynamic lady who spent a full weekend in a hotel room writing her purpose. It took her sixteen pages to fully express it. Through the next several years, she kept chipping away and refining those long sixteen pages. She finally got it down to eight words. Those eight words contained the essence of all that she wants to give to life, what she would like life to give back, and what she will become by playing out this possibility.

Your purpose must be created from deep soul-stirring questions:

- What am I?
- Who am I?
- How did I come into being?
- Why am I?
- Why am I here?
- What is my highest potential?
- If I fulfill my highest possible potential, what will I become?
- How do I fulfill that potential?
- Who am I to God?
- Who is God?
- Who is God to me?
- How can I come to know these things?

Try These Simple Questions:

- How do I show true love?
- How can I show more love?
- Do I express love plainly and frequently to my family and friends?
- What are my strengths?
- What are my weaknesses?
- How are my weaknesses really my strengths?
- How are my strengths really a sign of my weaknesses?
- Can I learn to love my weaknesses?
- Can I learn to use my strengths in a pure loving way?

By learning and developing your purpose, you will create a living testament to the value of this knowledge for your children. They will seek their own purpose because of the impact your example has had on their lives both directly and indirectly. They will naturally seek to emulate your progress. This may seem a little daunting to you at first. Just remember that you give your children an example to follow, good or bad. Try to make it the highest you have within you.

Our children will emulate the best and the worst in us. They will not emulate our possibility, but they will emulate our integrity and effort. They rarely will follow us into bland mediocrity. They will follow our most exceptional traits: the exceptionally good ones, as well as the bad ones. If we seek to improve both, we will lead them on a path through the delights of life. This can be an exciting quest through the mountain ranges of cause and effect on a grand universal scale.

Create a Mission Statement

After you come up with your purpose, create a broader statement called a mission statement. After you have formed your mission statement, come up with a vision. Then break your vision down into goals. Derive from the goal action statements called affirmations.

Chapter 30
The Nuts and Bolts of Purpose

If you wish to make an apple pie from scratch,
you must first invent the universe.
—Carl Sagan

Mission Statement: This is a brief statement of how we want to express our purpose in this mortal existence. How do you want to impact the world? How does your being here change the world for the better? This statement can and should fall fully within the bounds of mortality. It naturally grows out of your deepest cause. It contains all the aspects and intricacies expressed in your purpose. It will paint a more detailed picture of what life will be like living out your purpose.

Vision: This is where jobs, careers, fun, activities, passions, and opportunities are created and realized. It combines the depth of your purpose with the breadth of your mission and the iridescent color of your passions and loves. The vision is the image you have of how your life can fulfill the best possible scenario. It grows out of your purpose and is aligned with your mission.

Goals: Goals are where the rubber meets the road. This is where the purpose, mission, and vision are put into action. They are the defined objective that will result in the changes you want to see in your life. Make your goals measurable, time-oriented, and attainable. They must be a statement that leads to a specific action or behavior and results in a desired outcome. Goals have a time commitment. A goal not written is a wish at best. Write them down and read them every day. Half of your goals will be accomplished just by writing them down.

Affirmations: This is a delightful activity for you and your children. Next to your example, words are one of the most powerful teachers your children have. You will see a huge change take place in your life with the use of affirmations. An affirmation is a positive statement of fact, as it will be according to your goals, dreams, and most noble desires. State it in the present, as though it is already accomplished. State it in the positive as though it is already fact. Make affirmations short, powerful, reasonable, and attainable. Examples:

- I am lovable and loving.
- I am a genius and apply it in every situation.
- I am a great athlete and work hard for my success.
- I am an excellent student and learn out of desire for knowledge.
- I am good in every way.
- I am wise and use it to the benefit of all around me.
- I am a terrific parent.
- I am a kind and loving spouse.

Chapter 31
How Creative Are You?
Trouble is only opportunity in work clothes.
—Henry J. Kaiser

Remember, that which you vividly imagine and dwell upon will become your reality. What you think about, you bring about. As you contemplate and design your purpose, plan your mission, and integrate your vision with goals and actively use affirmations, you can become all that you believe yourself to be.

Keep your sights set high. Expect more. As you teach this to your children, they will be able to lengthen their stride to reach higher aims in life. Your children will be able to be confident without egotism, reach attainment without need of empty recognition, be effective and efficient, be able to love without the need to please, be relaxed in the midst of a busy life, and find peace in the rugged landscape of a tumultuous world.

1. Find your purpose by asking great questions. The quality of the questions you ask will determine the quality of your growth and thus your health.

2. Plan your mission. Make it concise and brief, but inclusive of your five big rocks.

3. Create your vision so it can sing to your soul.

4. Design goals that will lead you to your vision, mission, and purpose.

5. Create affirmations that detail the accomplishment of your goals. Your affirmations will attract to you the reality you choose.

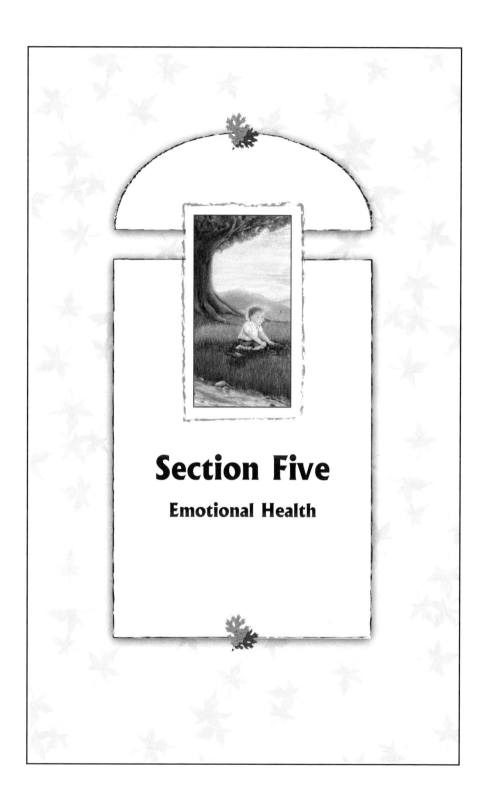

Section Five
Emotional Health

Chapter 32
Junk in, Junk Stays in

The first rule is to keep an untroubled spirit. The second is
to look things in the face and know them for what they are.
—Marcus Aurelius

Nutrition is often the dominant effort in many people's health plan. This is a critical part of good health. However, it can be a laborious way to regain lost health. Ponder for a moment what we put into our bodies more often than food. We drink usually more often than we eat. We breathe much more often than we eat or drink. Even more often than we breathe, we send thoughts to our body. Every thought has a physiological effect. Lie detector tests work on this premise. It has been said that the mind cannot tell the difference between a vividly imagined experience and a real event. The biggest difference is a real event only takes place one time. An imagined event usually gets re-experienced many times over in our mind. When we are in an experience, we do not go back and ponder about, worry over, or rethink it as it really happened. If we are creating our own reality of an experience, we will tend to rethink it and re-experience that situation over and over again in the context of our perception. It is probably not accurate and thus a myth. The experience, as we recall it, even though not real, has much greater impact on us than an authentic experience. One key to knowing how real you are during the experience is if you worried about it, have fear regarding it, or rethink that situation over repeatedly. If you revisit the event over and over again, you have not yet found the truth of it. In the Bible, this is called repentance. In modern terminology, we call it letting go. In reality, it is finding truth. Truth is always present. It remains constant in the past and the future, as well as in the present.

Thoughts create real and significant effects in our bodies. As a result, they have great effect on our health. How and what we think have great power over our health and our health potential. There is a relatively new branch of science called psychoneuroimmunology. It is the study of how our thoughts affect our immune system through our nerve system. Each thought causes the release of neurochemicals, or chemicals that affect our nerve system. Many of these neurochemicals go to all parts of our bodies. Immune cells have receptors for these chemicals that actually create emotions, as well as deep physical responses. One prominent scientist, Candace Pert, has stated that the "body is the subconscious mind." She believes that the body actually initiates thought by virtue of these molecules that dance back and forth between the brain cells and other body tissues and systems. The chemical serotonin is the focus of so much attention because it is involved in the pattern of behavior and thought we call depression and is also produced in the bowels as well as the heart. These organs can create emotion and respond to brain-induced emotional states. Bottom line: if you put junk into your body, in any way, food, air, or thought, it stays in and breeds. Give great care to your thoughts, self-talk and the attitude through which you view life.

Chapter 33
Emotions Are the Mirror of Spirituality

Living well and beautifully and justly are all one thing.
--Socrates

What are emotions? Emotions are the manifestations of our spiritual perspective as it touches our daily-perceived experiences. They are composed of four major parts:

1. Emotions can become learned reactions with a strong physical response.
2. Into this life we bring with us a nature and disposition that is an integral part of who we are: our true self, our spirit being. We have a mature and established nature as spirit beings. This is a formative part of our emotional disposition.
3. Our makeup is the spiritual perspective we develop as a philosophy during this stage of our existence.
4. We inherit a physical nature that carries many of the strong tendencies of our ancestors. As we seek to improve ourselves, these characteristics can also be channeled in a positive direction.

Chapter 34
Reaction: The Breakfast of Victims

All learning is recollection.
--Plato

As our spiritual perspective is based in reality, reality being God's perspective, and through this perspective, we will enjoy peace and power in life. In every circumstance, there is a highest reality, a representation of things as they really exist. This view is God's view. When we see things the way God sees things, we are based in a powerful spiritual reality. When we see things this way, we begin to see life on the physical plane differently. Some may ask, "Is this possible?" In the book of 1 John 3:2 it says: "When he shall appear, we shall be like him; for we shall see him as he is."

When we see things the way God sees things, we will become all we can become. Then we will see ourselves as we really are, and others the way God sees them. The more we are aware of our true nature, why we are here in this life, and where we are going, the better able we are to act and not react. As long as we maintain the divinely bestowed right to choose, we are able to act. To act means we are not a victim but a cause. As soon as we choose to react, to anything or anyone, we lose our authentic power and become a victim and not a cause. We become a victim not of the situation but of our choice to be ruled by the circumstance. When we become a victim, we lose the power to choose. There are emotions of action and emotions of reaction. The emotions of action are healthy. The emotions of reaction are negative and do not have a positive effect on our health in either length of life or quality of life.

When we act, we act out of love. As soon as we react, we respond out of judgment. When we judge, we are acting based on our limited perception of what we think just happened. Of one thing we can be sure. We will never know exactly what another is thinking by watching their actions. As a result, our response, if based on what we think they were thinking, would be flawed and self-centered. It will be based on anger, fear, or their ugly brother, worry. We will be trying to create an outcome we think is right. We may try to make others happy. We may try to make them sad. We may try and remove the stress we think they have. But we really have no power in anyone outside of being loving.

Each day in life we face choices. Every interaction with another person leads to a chance to face reality or to remain in your current perception of it. If we see the person in each experience as God sees them, we will have a deep understanding of other's needs and the motives behind individual choices. This is why Stephen Covey teaches: "Seek first to understand, then to be understood." If we can be sure we understand our children, spouse, or friend, our interaction is based in a common reality and communication can occur. The very word communication is based on the word 'common'. We can only communicate if we have a common understanding. If we react, we have no common ground with our children.

A patient once shared the frustration of a son who had suddenly stopped doing his homework in a critical class. He was striving to be accepted into a very prestigious private school. At a critical time in the application, interview process he stopped applying himself in one specific class. Then he started hanging out with a very different peer group. Both parents were frustrated. They tried threatening, scolding and bribing him to do better. During a visit to my office I asked the mother a pointed question, "What is more important to you. . . your son or his admission into the private school?" She responded that obviously it was her son. I encouraged her to make sure he knew that. The light of understanding turned on. She went home that night and at the right moment expressed to her son that she loved him and that he was more important to her than any behavior, school or grade. If he made it into the school or not, it didn't matter to her. He was incredible in her eyes no matter what he chose to do. She communicated her feelings with such integrity that he instantly believed her. Tears of gratitude filled his eyes and he hugged her. They wept together. She honored her statement to him by not pushing him any more about his classes. His response was to catch up on his homework, pick up his studies, and recapture his previous level of performance.

He needed to know that he was more important than his performance or accomplishment. His parents were reacting and feeling victimized by his poor choices. When his mother started to act out of her real feelings, her love for her son, he was freed of great pressure and expectation and able to be himself.

When we see things as they really are, we are always powerful. Only when we react to our judgment of others do we become a victim and thus powerless.

Chapter 35
Chaos Versus Order

Fear of misfortune is worse than misfortune itself.
—Najile S. Khoury

Emotions create physical responses. Fear is a foundational emotion. It is the precursor to many other emotions, nearly all of them negative. Fear and love are creative emotions. Fear creates chaos, and love creates order. That which we fear we materialize in our life. That which we fear we create in greater and greater levels of chaos. That which we love we create in greater and greater levels of order. If a person is afraid of something, he will attract that thing into his life. If he loves something, he will attract that thing into his life. This is why insurance companies raise rates on a person who has an accident. They know if an individual has one, the next is usually not far behind. They know that one leads to more. They raise the rates to adapt ahead of time to what experience has taught them will transpire.

If you have an unpleasant occurrence in life, you would be wise to ask, "How did I attract that into my life?" Learn the lesson before it must be repeated.

I believe there are ultimately two emotions: fear and its derivations, and love with its associated virtues. If you want to know your deepest emotional state, look at what you have attracted into your life. It is that which you love or that which you fear. If you love your life, you are acting out of love. If you are not pleased with your life, you are acting out of fear at some level.

Love Is a Choice

Emotions of action are those emotions based in virtue. These emotions are founded on the virtue of love. Love is a choice and a mindset we actively choose. Love is also a state, or a way of being, that is a gift from God. It is a way of looking at things "as they really are." Love is the view of life from a divine lens. Love is never manipulative and does not require others to behave a certain way for free and full expression. If we need our children to behave a certain way for us to love them, we are manipulating, not loving. In this case, our children would have an unspoken responsibility to behave a certain way so we can be comfortable. This type of comfort is rarely virtuous.

Love is not judgmental, but it is consistent. You can love and still have rules and guidelines. Love is just. As a result it has consequences, but it is never arbitrary. Favors and freedoms are hinged on actions, and there are set consequences to those actions. We can deliver appropriate consequences and still love. In fact, it is almost impossible to love without some level of justice. All people need guidelines to grow by. Transgressions of these guidelines must result in consequences. If we act out of wisdom, we will choose appropriate consequences. The best consequences are rarely harsh and usually result in the transgressor and you, the judge, feeling more kindly to one another. The result of justice is always the optimal opportunity of growth for both parties.

By mindfully choosing our motivation, love or fear, we will create a powerful example in life for our children to emulate. As we are consistent in our example of love, our children will choose to pattern our example. A feeble and aging grandmother lived with her daughter and granddaughter. As she grew frail, she frequently dropped plates, spilled water and created far more mess than she could help clean up. One day, exasperated because the old woman had broken another prized plate, the daughter sent the granddaughter to buy the grandmother a wooden plate. The granddaughter hesitated because she knew a wooden plate would humiliate the elderly woman. But, her mother insisted, so reluctantly she went to the store. She returned with two wooden plates. "I only asked you to buy one," the mother said. "Why have you purchased two?" I bought one for grandmother now" she responded, "And I bought one, Mother, for you when you get old."

Check yourself consistently:

- Do I act out of fear or out of love?
- Do I have a specific outcome in mind?
- Am I manipulating or loving?

Your children will emulate you. Try to be mindful of your motives and the inevitable outcomes.

Chapter 36
Living in the Present

We are what we are, wherever we are.
—Richard L. Evans

Love resides only in the present moment. If we see our children's behavior and worry about what others will think, we are not acting out of love. By creating in our mind other people's possible reactions, we are transporting ourselves into an imaginary future based on our assumptions of what we think others will think. An old saying goes, "It doesn't matter what I think, and it doesn't matter what you think. What matters is what I think you think." As soon as we make an assumption or judge another, we are dealing in our imagined reality, one of which the other person has no concept. Nothing will ever happen as we have imagined it. As we start to make assumptions about the future or the past, love cannot exist in us. Love only dwells in the moment we are currently living.

If we worry about the past or fear the future, we wander aimlessly, trapped in imaginary states of our own creation that will never exist in reality but only in our own minds. If we use the emotions of anger, fear, worry, frustration, or any of their inbred cousins, we are not living in the present nor are we living out of love.

There are three realities that exist, with which we must deal. There is our own reality, the world as we see it. Then, there is the reality of others. They have very different experiences than we do even in the same circumstances in the same time and place. The third reality is that of God. The closer our view becomes like God's, the more we are living in reality and out of love. In that view, we can see more clearly the motives others have. We can see them more as they really are. Try and look at any circumstance from the same view God has. If your child talks back to you, how does God see that situation? How can you shift your view to match God's view? Is your attitude one of love? What is your child's view? Is he in a more correct view of things than you are? When you can see things as they really are, then you are getting close. If you are having a hard time seeing any other perspective than your own, it is an indication you are not healthy in your view.

When I was young, I had done something that was wrong. I had broken a window throwing a rock at my brother. My only regret was that I had missed him. I knew it was wrong, and my father knew it. I just did not want to admit I had made a mistake. He had teased me in a way that I let get under my skin. I was still angry about his teasing me. I guess I thought I could do something unacceptable with no consequences. My father talked to me, but I still refused to accept responsibility. Finally, seeing he wasn't making any headway talking to me, my father removed his belt. I was shocked. He had never done that before.

I had heard about this type of thing, but I had never been struck with a belt. I was a little frightened. He said that if I did not see that something wrong had been done, then someone else needed to be punished for my wrong action.

He then gave me the belt, laid his hand on the table next to me, and told me to hit his hand with the belt. I told him I did not want to hit him. He said someone should be punished for the misdeed. If he had not taught me any better than that, then he should be punished. I cried and told him I did not want to hit him. He persisted, and I cried more. He insisted until I had feebly struck his hand a few times. He was patient and loving, and taught a valuable lesson. I never tried to "duck" the consequences of my actions after that event. I also realized how much I loved my father and would never want to hurt him. Wisdom combined with love is the best teacher.

My father's focus was on me. He was interested in my well-being and education. He was not concerned with perception, power, or control. He was interested in me learning a lesson. He was willing to take a whipping to let me learn. He was fully present with me that day.

Love, peace, joy, learning, discovering truth, and the experience of God in our lives comes only through living in the moment. As soon as we leave the present moment, we leave all possibility of finding any virtuous state.

Excellent Parenting

Learning to be present with our children is a major key to excellence in parenting. Being a parent means we must take full responsibility in demonstrating virtues our children can emulate. As we refine and demonstrate virtue in our lives, our children will be attracted to the example. Genuine laughter comes from being in the present. When you can laugh at yourself or at your children's mistakes, you are much closer to the reality and the present.

Anger or frustration indicates we are slipping out of the present and acting from a past experience. This will ensure we do not communicate the love we feel for our children. It will withdraw our ability to act. We begin to react to an imaginary view of reality that we have created in our own minds. It does not exist in anyone else's reality. It is a myth. When we are living in this false state, we feel unappreciated, misunderstood, and unloved. When we are in a false state, our children usually feel misunderstood. They have trust in us, but all of their considerable instincts clash with our actions and motivations. This is when children lose trust in us. They know something is more important to us than they are. They begin to realize we are not powerful enough to continue to teach them. Often they are right. Regain your power by refusing to react. Choose to act and to respond out of virtue, not out of circumstance.

I heard a story of a woman who was shopping one day in a department store. A clearance sale was taking place. Next to her was a young mother who was much more intent on the clothing than on her toddler. The child had become impatient with the prolonged sifting through clothes, seeking that great buy. The child had no value in her mother's interest. She was feeling less than important. By complaining she let her mother know she was not happy about being second fiddle. The mother responded impatiently at being interrupted. The child persisted loudly.

She wanted to go. Finally, the mother reacted aggressively. The woman watching this interchange felt she could not watch the mother treat her child so roughly. She was about to turn away and walk to another area of the store but strongly felt she needed to intercede. She tried to walk away but found herself turning around, walking right up to the young mother and saying, "You have a beautiful young daughter. Can I talk to her?"

The mother, stiff and defensive at first, quickly relented. They both knelt down and talked to the bright and beautiful child. The mother's heart was softened, turned to love and away from her self-centered distraction. The mother and daughter were at peace again. Reality was restored. The mother reconnected to the present. Only when she started acting out of her real value did she feel the love she had for her daughter.

Chapter 37
Activities for Present Living

A wise man will make more opportunities than he finds.
—Francis Bacon

How do we integrate activities that help to teach ourselves and our families to be in the present?

Listen to your children. Much of their self-worth is based on how important their feelings and experiences are to you as a parent. Listen to their words, but listen most especially to why they need to talk. This is critical when you are busy. Try to never disregard their needs. The more they are ignored, the more they will need to be heard, and the more they will act out. Hear what a child needs to express when he talks. Very often, he needs to satisfy an unexpressed need. It is not his words that are important; it is the feelings that initiate the words. If we don't hear him, he will find someone who will listen, even if it is an unhealthy peer.

When a child is hurt and cries, avoid the tendency to shush her. Let her cry it out. It will help her to process the event and eliminate the pent up energy of the trauma. Once the energy and emotion of the trauma are relieved, the experience can be correctly categorized in her life encyclopedia. All our future decisions come from the writings in this life encyclopedia. If we shush them and stop the needed expression of the pent up emotions of the trauma, they carry that energy in them to be expelled at some later inappropriate time.

One night, one of my daughters, age eleven, seemed particularly upset. I asked her if something was wrong. She responded briefly that it was friend problems. Sensing that she was not going to talk but needed to express her feelings, I sat down next to her on the floor and asked her if she needed to cry. She said, "probably." I asked her if I could hold her while she cried. She said, "Okay." She leaned over and rested on my shoulder. I put my arm around her and held her head as she started to cry. She cried for about ten minutes. Suddenly, she stopped, sat up straight, and said, "I'm done." I was excused. She felt better. In fact, she has dealt with friend problems much better ever since. She just needed a safe place to express her emotion.

Retain the power of choice

Help teach your children the power of being able to choose their response in any situation. We cannot control our circumstances, but we can always benefit from them. Help your children see the various ways to look at situations. If it is difficult to understand why the other person would act the way he does, put yourself in his or her place. Imagine what he might be feeling that might cause him to behave in that way. If you still cannot understand, change what you think his emotions seemed to be to some other emotional state. Ask the questions: If he were afraid, why would he act this way? If he were sad, why would he choose this behavior? Keep trying other emotions until you no longer find negativity in the situation. If he were frightened, could it cause him to act this way? What could frighten someone in such a way? What did you feel when you were with him? Remember that anger is always a derivative of fear. Try and walk a mile in his shoes. Always find the way to maintain your power of choice and the power to act in every situation. When we see other people as they really are, instead of the way we choose to see them, we are empowered to act out of our own strengths and powers. If we are reacting to others, we are either trying to manipulate them to regain control, or we are letting them control us. In Chinese language, the written word for crisis and opportunity is the same character. Help your children practice the recognition of their personal power of choice by acting and not reacting in all situations.

Be respectful of others' space, time, choices, and needs

Judging others is the easiest path and serves our biggest weaknesses. Help your children to seek the good in every person and in every situation. Find words that express respect for others' choices rather than criticism for their differences. It is a better person who sees the virtue or the pain, rather than the flaws behind another's choices.

One young woman, whose father was brutally murdered by a group of young men, struggled with the intense emotions of loss and the apparent prejudice behind the violence. Some time later she received a letter from one of the men who killed her father. He apologized, begged her forgiveness, and recounted to her the story of his life, filled with abuse of every kind since childhood. He told of his search for himself gone wild. He had not realized he had become exactly what he had learned to hate as a child, violence. Once the woman saw the pain in the young man associated with her father's death, her entire outlook changed. She shifted from being a victim to being an advocate of change. Be wise enough to see behind the action to the person who acted. Be sure enough of yourself to see what pain others may carry that causes them to act out in violence.

Refuse to criticize

Criticism is easy and simply reinforces our own weaknesses. Recognize that everyone is smart, beautiful, good, and incredible in individual ways. When we criticize, it is a sign we are unwilling to see virtue. It is only difficult to see the virtue in another if you cannot see your own virtue in that circumstance. Research has shown that our criticism is not a reflection of others but of ourselves. Let us assume the responsibility to see our own virtue. When we can see ourselves in an honest way, with kind eyes and a forgiving attitude, we are free to see others in the same way, as they really are. If you criticize someone, you are viewed by those you are speaking to as having the same fault you are accusing the absent party of having. If you speak positively of a person in his absence, you are seen as having the same virtue. If you call someone a good athlete in his absence, others view you as being a good athlete. We are judged in the same manner we judge. The Bible teaches this principle, "For with what judgment ye judge, so shall ye also be judged."

Learn how to ask so you can receive

The Bible teaches, "Ask and ye shall receive. Knock and it shall be open unto you." If we do not ask, we will not get. Does it ever hurt to ask? If we do not ask, the only answer can be no. Only if we ask can we receive what we desire. These guidelines apply to asking of God, as well as others.

Critical Ingredients to Successful Asking

1. Create the right intent. Ask for the right thing for the right reason.
2. Know the universe as God has created it is abundant. If you get what you ask for, it does not mean that another will lack.
3. Know how to ask. Be direct and humble.
4. Expect to receive.
5. Be willing to accept whatever God will give as abundance.
6. Reaffirm the eventual with accepting affirmations beforehand.
7. Have an attitude of gratitude on asking. Believe you will receive. Be grateful for any outcome.

This pattern works in prayer and with asking things of others. Ask. You cannot fail unless you do not ask. If you are in a store to purchase an item, ask a sales person, "Is this your best price?" It cannot hurt. If he can lower the price, you save.

If not, you do not lose anything. With your spouse, ask directly for what you want. With your children learn to be direct in your requests of them.

Serve others' needs with no expectation of response. Selfless service will bring joy and awareness to life that will increase your child's spiritual and emotional strength. Do not give with expectation to "get" something in return. Give to give, and you will always receive in abundance. The Tao de Ching, the Taoists book of spiritual philosophy, says, "Do your work with no thought of outcome." If we serve out of authentic concern, we will open the back door of our soul to the cascading abundance of the universe. One excellent way to access these blessings is to start your children out young teaching them the benefits of tithing. A tithe is a return of one tenth of your increase to God who gave you all you have. Malachi, in the Bible teaches, "[I will] open you the windows of heaven, and pour you out a blessing, that [there shall] not [be room] enough [to receive it]." Find a worthy group to give your tithe. By giving back to God one tenth with the intention of gratitude, you will never lack. You can give to a church, charity, or organization that serves a virtuous cause. This will open the windows of your soul to the universal fountain of cause.

Recognize God created the universe on principles of abundance not on scarcity. The universe was created on the basis of absolute abundance. The only time there is a lack in the universe is when we introduce it. The universe is brimming with possibilities of an endless nature. Teach your children that by accessing the right behaviors and intentions, the heavens will open. Asking how big is your piece of the "pie" is an improper question. A better question is "How big is the "pie"? The "pie" of life extends beyond the broadest horizons of our imagination. It is infinite, and anything is possible. The universe is built of an endless array of resources, and from it we can build anything. All the pieces are there. We can build any attitude, object, or life we can imagine. We just need to believe in ourselves and the power God has allowed each of us. When I was young, my parents taught me I could do anything I wanted to in life and could become whatever I chose as long as I followed the laws established as guardians of those realities. They were, and are, correct.

Chapter 38
Free To Be Me

Children are like spaghetti; you can pull them
but you cannot push them.
—Author unknown

Be aware of how your children act around different individuals. Children are sometimes uncomfortable around certain people. Honor their right to feel that way. Do not force them to be window dressing for your social standing. Children act out for good reasons. At a later, peaceful time, ask them how they felt when they were uncomfortable. If they are having a hard time explaining their feelings, encourage them to use colors, animals, weather, textures, tastes, or smells to describe the way they felt about the person they wanted to avoid.

If a child's awareness is different from the parents', expressing his feelings and perceptions may be difficult. If the child does not like being around a certain adult or relative, it does not mean the person is bad, just that the child does not feel good with that individual. Excuse the child from the situation, and encourage coloring a picture about the way he felt in that situation. This helps to express feelings and aids understanding.

Then help the child understand the power of choice. S e e i n g many options, allows the situation to become empowering. Many children have sensitivities their parents do not possess. Ignoring the child's perceptions can cause a deep self-distrust in your child, resulting in low self-esteem and seemingly errat-ic patterns of behavior.

If a child seems impossible to reach, it is often because par-ents have not yet found the right way to listen or interact with him. Children often have different personality styles than their parents. Because of this, they do not learn the traits and pat-terns necessary to use and access their gifts and abilities. We learn from the amazing work in neurolinguistic programming that people manifest their inner dialogues by their physiologi-cal patterns of behavior. If we want to feel what someone else is feeling, we can copy their physical patterns, and we will feel very much what they feel. If our personality style is very differ-ent from theirs, it can be very uncomfortable to mimic their physical patterns. It will create a lot of tension inside. This is what happens to many children. They mimic the behavior of their parents so closely that they feel what their parents feel. These feelings can be so foreign to the nature of the child that it is like a cold front and a warm front coming together. This can spark emotional thunderstorms inside a child that will spill out in their behavior.

Chapter 39
Who Are You Anyway?

"Trailing clouds of glory do we come,
from God who is our home."
—William Wordsworth

Children are wonderful, amazing, pure, and open. They are not, however, simple. The more aware a parent is of her children's true nature and emotions, the more she helps meet their needs. The more children know parents are aware and not condemning of their feelings, the more they will let parents inside their heads and hearts. You can help them be accepting of these emotions. Many children see the incongruity in the parents' emotions and cannot understand the reason for it. They will often withdraw from the parent because of this.

Another reaction children often have when they are different from their parents is to believe there is something wrong inside of them. Children have to be very strong to be different than either parent and still feel good about themselves. If you have a child who seemed to come from another planet, be aware. Do not expect him to comply with your attitudes, likes, and dislikes. Expect virtuous choices, but realize they may be different than yours. Celebrate their uniqueness. If we insist he be like us, the child's self-esteem may starve, and he will have many of the problems related to the oft-described state of low self-esteem. Allow your children to be different from you in their emotions and reactions. Encourage it. Let them know that they are not bad just because they feel differently than you do. You can tell them this, but it is infinitely better to show them by being present with them. Be with them consistently enough that they feel your acceptance. They will know that they are okay even if they are different than you. Be content with the goodness of your child and their virtue rather than a set pattern of behavior.

Values of virtue are not optional in this context. Virtues are to be abided in all situations. Remember, expressions like crying are not un-virtuous. Make sure you understand the child well enough to know that he or she may be honest, but that the child may see situations differently than you see them. Allow him to see situations differently than you. Recognize his honesty has little to do with your perception. Children have different experiences than we have. Allow them to see things differently and discuss the differences. Both you and your child will learn. Keep the virtuous path, and your children will be attracted to it.

If your children are like you, celebrate inside, for they are easier to understand. But if not, be accepting nonetheless. How will our children ever exceed us if we do not let them be different than we are?

Chapter 40
Strategies for Emotional Balance

God sells us all things at the price of labor.
—Leonardo da Vinci

Practice balance in judgment. If you catch yourself or your children commenting negatively about someone or something, employ the positive three game: state three good things about that person or thing within the next minute.

Pattern for connection. When listening to your child, match his body posture and breathing pattern. Listen intently without judging what he says. Ask him back, "Is this what you are trying to say?" or "Am I hearing correctly?"

Affirmations. Use words that reflect abundance. Instead of saying, "We can't afford that," you might say, "How can you afford this? When you want to start I will help you" or "That sounds worth working for. How do you think you could earn that?"

Encourage expression. Let your children express their emotions in a traumatic situation. Let them cry it out all the way.

Do not shush them; it is a critical part of processing the ener-gy from the trauma. When children suppress energy of trauma, it will likely be expressed in the body or behavior. Emotional honesty is a key to happiness. Accept responsibility for your own feelings. Teach your children the same trait. Emotions relate strongly to spiritual perspective. Our emotions are the by-product of our spiritual perspective as it combines with our life experiences. Link the emotions to the corresponding spiri-tual perspective with emotions as a guide. Work to strengthen their spiritual perspective. If a child believes even God cannot love them, it will manifest in their emotional make up. Use emo-tions as a way to back track to understand the spiritual view of the child.

Creative expression. Encourage a free expression of creative thoughts and feelings. Help your children express their feelings artistically. Talk to them about their art and what it feels like to them.

Musical expression. Music opens up the heart. Help your children find music that helps them express themselves. Listening is almost as good as performing. Make sure the music is uplifting. As clearly demonstrated in the book, *The Secret Life of Plants*, even plants do not like anger-motivated music. Our children will be more relaxed and peaceful as you select good music. Research also shows children learn better with the influence of classical music.

Our children will be more relaxed and peaceful as we select good music. Research discussed in EurekaAlert, a web based information site, of March 23, 2004, teaches that children who listen to music while exercising boost their brainpower. Sharlene Habermeyer elaborates on this powerful resource in her great book, *Good Music, Brighter Children*.

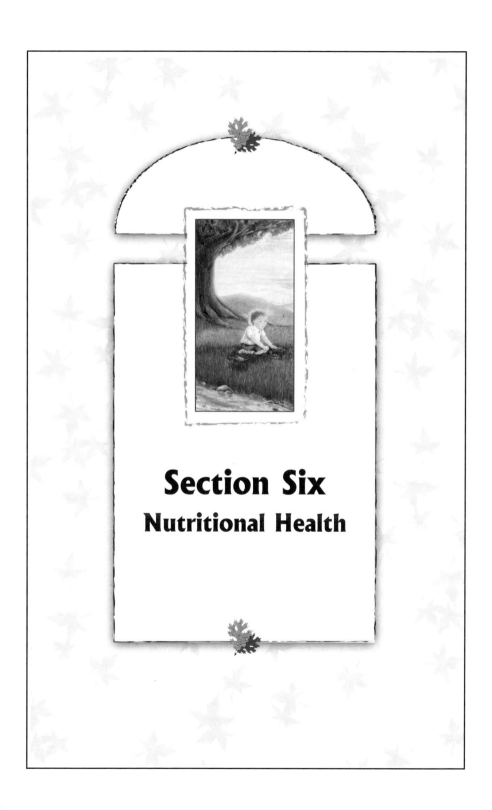

Section Six
Nutritional Health

Chapter 41
If We Eat It, We Will Be It

Few seem conscious that there is such a thing
as physical morality.
—Herbert Spencer

As the old song teaches, "What goes up must come down." In nutrition, "What goes in must come out." It comes out in what our body emanates, as well as what our body eliminates. What we eat is manifest in what our body radiates. It is manifest in our complexion, endurance, strength, self-control, quality of our body tissue and cells, and the sparkle in our eyes. What we consume is one of the main determiners of what we put out in thought, action, and in what we feel. If a person drinks alcohol, it has a cumulative effect, and his behavior is altered even after the alcohol wears off. What we put in our mouths will have some effect at some point on the quality of our lives as a whole.

The physical body we inhabit is a product of nature and is the means our spirit has to express itself. The nurture and care given to the body will manifest itself in the clarity of our spiritual expression. Thus, the things we put into our bodies become immediately reflected in the clarity of our spiritual experience. If a person uses drugs, either prescription or illegal, to numb feelings or to escape circumstances, the individual loses the opportunity to gain insight of a spiritual nature from those situations. What we put into our bodies will rarely be neutral in effect. Nutrition either enhances our clarity of being, or it will cloud the spiritual lens through which we see life. It will either enable us to clearly understand the feelings our bodies send us or cloud the delicate, spiritual senses that are so important in personal growth and vibrant health. Good nutrition will help us comprehend ourselves in our environment. Good nutrition provides clean nutrients with little to no chemical or energetic static. The static created in the body from poor nutritional habits, like the static on a radio, will cloud the body's ability to:

- Respond to its constant need to rebuild itself
- Express itself
- Maintain balance and self-awareness by creating false messages that will mislead the body in its efforts.

Nutrition provides the building blocks from which our body will rebuild itself on nearly an annual basis. Our body has nearly 60 trillion cells. We are constantly constructing new replacement cells to keep our tissue new and strong. Our body makes in the vicinity of two hundred fifty thousand new cells per second. Children grow and develop so quickly. Providing good nutrition is vital for their well being.

Chapter 42
The Gentle Current of Nutrition

Life is not a goblet to be drained;
it is a measure to be filled.
—Author unknown

Nutrition is a critical part of nurturing our body, mind, and spirit. There are definite spiritual, emotional, and physical consequences to what we put into our bodies. Recreational drugs definitely have negative consequences. How can something like marijuana, which kills brain cells, not have a deep emotional and spiritually clouding effect? Many prescription drugs also have a fog-like effect on our spiritual perceptions. Every prescription medication has side effects. Even if the side effects do not reach a clinical level of manifestation, like showing up on a blood test as liver damage, they will still have a subtle impact on the cleaning function of the liver. If any substance has a physical effect, it will have a more powerful effect on our more delicate, emotional system and on the infinitely more delicate sensitivities of our spiritual awareness. How does a child's diet impact behavior?

From experience I know what children consume has a vast

impact on their ability to express themselves but also on their ability to understand themselves. Many children experience frustration because of the emotions they feel after eating certain foods that we call treats. We proclaim the snack good, but the child feels bad after eating it. It is a difficult thing for the child to understand and comprehend. He feels bad after he eats something we call "good." This forms one more contradiction they must distort themselves to fit into.

Food has a more gentle effect than drugs on our emotions, energy level, and ability to gain access to our spiritual senses, but a consistent effect, nonetheless. Anything we take into our body that creates a buzz, like caffeine, the release of alcohol, or the feeling or nurture from sweets, will cloud the gentle and delicate spiritual promptings we must learn to feel and follow to realize our highest potential. The path to the highest that is within us is a narrow, rocky ridge-riding trail with often-precipitous sides. It is a path often concealed by erosion of junk food, unneeded medication, recreational alcohol, and drugs. These make the path to our highest potential hard to find and follow.

Make Wise Food Choices

I am not suggesting that we have to eat perfectly for good health, but we must use wisdom in our choices of foods. An occasional treat is good for the soul, but abuses of sweets, refined foods, alcohol, drugs, or stimulants can cause an emotional, physical, and or spiritual dependence that clouds our view of "reality." We soon begin to nurture this self-created mythical view of life and ourselves with more unbalancing nutritional choices. We develop the need to sustain our comfort zones rather than the divine inner voice. In these patterns of behavior, although self-destructive, we find the comfort of familiarity. The unknown path of self-awareness is usually more frightening than the known pathway of pain.

A storied king in the Middle Ages would place an undesirable visitor in an arena to choose his destiny. The prisoner was placed before two gates and told to choose one. Behind one gate they were informed was a lion and sure death. Behind the other gate was an unknown fate. They had to choose one of the gates. Three of four prisoners chose the lion. The thought of choosing the unknown was worse than choosing sure death. The known death was preferred to the possibility of freedom, which is exactly what awaited them behind the unknown gate.

Chapter 43
Nutrition Made Incredibly Easy

There is more to life than increasing its speed.
-—Mahatma Ghandi

Good nutrition is very simple. It is made up of three main parts:

Nutrition is the process of transferring energy from the sun to your body. Through photosynthesis, the plant kingdom transfers the energy of pure light to caloric energy found in food. The closer the food is to the source, the sun, the more nurturing light the food possesses. The more light it has, the more life it gives. A fresh piece of fruit from the tree is very good. Canned fruit is not as good as a piece of fresh fruit because it is further removed from light. A fruit pie does not have as much life energy as does the fresh fruit and so on down the chain. The more food is processed the less benefit we gain.

Eat food that grows in the climate in which we live, in the season that it grows. If you live in northern areas, eat the food grown by local gardeners in the season that it grows. In winter months when nothing grows, eat foods that store well like grains, beans, potatoes, onions, carrots, meats, etc. Foods naturally contain the energy and nutrition to balance us with the climate.

Choose food that is clean. Clean food is organic or as unaltered as possible. The fewer the pesticides and artificial fertilizers, the better the food is for you. Good choices are meats that are fed on nature's food. Cattle should be fed on grass. Chicken and turkey should be free range, meaning they eat what they want out of nature, not the manufactured feed commonly fed them. Eat fresh fish from the natural environment, not farm raised. They are healthier. Milk is most nutritious unpasteurized and from grass-fed cows. We should eat most of our food according to this pattern. As we eat from these guidelines, we avoid the traps of food-induced conditions like high blood pressure, high cholesterol, obesity and all the subsequent illnesses and receive all the benefits nature intended.

Eat to:
- Gain good wholesome nutrition
- Achieve balance with the seasons
- Allow free expression of your spiritual nature

Eating to satisfy our appetites or emotional needs will lead us down winding paths that inevitably lead to the problems mentioned above.

This simple approach will cover all three aspects thoroughly. Rigid compliance is not needed. A sincere effort to apply these concepts will create an inner change in your heart and mind. The benefits will reach inside your innermost being. As you receive these benefits, your children will observe the effects and mimic them. Your good habits will become your children's good habits, creating benefit at every level.

Another area of serious concern that requires awareness is foods that are stimulants or sedatives, like coffee, alcohol, soda pop, chocolate, sugar-laden foods, and dietary or symptom-based herbal blends. These should be used with great caution. They are foods that create wide swings in our physical, emotional, and spiritual pendulum. Our bodies must go through chemical gymnastics to accommodate these foods and their potent effects. The belief that these items are helpful is born out of emotional dishonesty. If you do not have the energy to get out of bed in the morning without your coffee, you must consider your health, or lack of it, and why this would be. If any of these become a consistently used crutch, look at the emotions or physical causes that may underlie their use. Seek to create balance with the emotions, physical, or spiritual need and not to rely on the addiction of choice. As always, realize that the examples you show your children will strongly influence their behavior. As you find the core causes underlying your choices and balance their effects in your life, you will be better able to effectively relate with your children.

Chapter 44
The Problem Rests Within

"The root of the matter is found in me."
Job 19:28

I remember a presentation I gave to a civic organization several years back. The topic was on the drug problem in our country. I was just getting started when one of the senior members interrupted me and asked, "We are all aware of the problem, so what is the solution." He definitely caught me unaware. I looked at him as he held a cigarette in one hand and his third pre-lunch alcoholic drink in the other and noticed the same state in most of the other attendees. I wanted to say, "You are the problem. Look how you are handling your stress. How can our kids choose otherwise?" I am saddened to admit I tanked. I hedged and did not come right out and state that "we" are the problem. How could we expect our children to make healthy choices when they have witnessed our example and dependence on these substances? As soon as they get stressed, they are going to do what they have seen, look for something to help them cope. They may use recreational drugs or the common drugs of sugar, alcohol, tobacco, and stimulants like caffeine. They may use prescription drugs to hide from the real issues that dwell in the cellars of our body, mind, and soul. Children do what they see us do, cope through chemistry and food rather than deal with the realities of life. Thus, we create the drug problem in our country from the drugs of alcohol, tobacco, and misuse of prescription drugs.

Food is the second leading cause of health problems in our society. If we choose our nutritional habits wisely, we will not only avoid the pitfalls but also enjoy the increased levels of wellness that can come from easy dietary upgrades.

Fruits are an excellent snack food. Blueberries have more antioxidants that help prevent cancer and wrinkles than any other food we know of. Other berries and fruits are powerful nutrition, and easy to get kids to eat.

Include plenty of vegetables. They are great sources of healthy nutrition. For solutions to picky vegetable eaters see www.ChildrenofPromise.net.

A healthy balance of meat is proper nutrition. I encourage free-range chicken, grass-fed beef, freshwater fish from a clean stream, or ocean fish caught far from the shore and industrialization. Supplementing omega-3 fats is a good idea if you can't include healthy fish every two weeks.

Clean water: if you do not drink filtered water, you are the filter. Please find a way to get your family clean drinking water. You can get a home filter for pennies a day. See www.ChildrenofPromise.net for information on how to get clean water.

Beans are the forgotten miracle food. They sustain health, fight disease, are easy to prepare, and most people like them.

Whole grains get a bad rap from some people. I believe whole grains to be very healthy. The fresher the better.

Refined carbohydrates are a problem for anyone and should generally be avoided. Whole grains in breads, cooked cereals, and pastas are very acceptable in good nutrition.

Nuts and seeds are nutritious snacks. They are a must on salads and a great after-school snack.

Chapter 45
Do as I Do, Not as I Say

My life is my message.
—Mahatma Ghandi

As we create health from a positive place of desire and passion, we naturally seek a balanced lifestyle by positive intention with a firm grasp on the desired outcome. If we live life with the goal of vibrant health in all its characteristics as the objective, we will likely achieve that objective. If we live life hoping to avoid disease, at best we will delay the inevitable onset of disease, but we can never encounter a truly healthy existence. We will hamper the full enjoyment of our daily life, and our ability to express our full potential will be limited. We will neither experience the abundant joy this life has to offer or share with others the full measure of our truest nature.

As we choose good food, our energy will improve, our immune function will be effective, our mind will be active and quick, our muscles will be more pliable, and our joints will be more flexible and less likely to inflame in the agony of chronic arthritis. A clean diet will clean the blood and help the bowels stay active and effective in cleansing the body. Our urinary system will be less subject to infections. The liver will not get overburdened with its thousands of functions. Our hormone balance will improve. There is no system in the body that will not be improved with a clean and nutritious diet.

A mother once traveled a great distance to bring her son to see Gandhi. After their long and difficult journey, they stood in line for some time to see the famous spiritual leader. When they were finally brought before the great man, Gandhi asked, "What can I do for you?" The mother responded, "Will you please tell my son to stop eating sugar? It is very bad for him, and he will not stop eating sugar. I love him, and I know it is bad for him, but he will not stop eating sugar. Will you tell him to stop? I know he will listen to you." Gandhi looked at the boy for a moment, and then he turned to the mother and said, "Go away. Come back in two weeks." "But we have traveled so far. We have stood in line most of the day," replied the mother.

"Go away and come back in two weeks." Gandhi said. So, the mother and son left and returned in two weeks. After the long day's travel and another long wait in line, the mother and boy were finally again before Gandhi. "Two weeks ago we traveled all this way to see you. I asked you to tell my son to stop eating sugar. You told us to go away and come back in two weeks. Well, here we are," said the mother. Gandhi looked at her and then at the boy. He held his finger out in front of the boy, and shaking it he said "Young man, I want you to stop eating sugar. It is not good for you." The young man instantly looked more humbled and replied, "Yes sir. I won't eat sugar any more." The mother was shocked. "Why didn't you do that two weeks ago? We have had to travel so far. Why not just tell him this same thing when we were here two weeks ago?" "Two weeks ago" said Gandhi "I was eating sugar."

If there is a problem with the fruit of a tree, always look first to the roots. As you go through this book, it will be important for you to make changes in your life, even if they are small and simple. As you do this, your children will naturally assimilate the changes you have made into their own lives. As you work with your children, you will be working with them out of a place of virtue and integrity. They will feel the difference in the message just the way Gandhi knew the boy would sense his lack of integrity if he told the boy to stop eating sugar, which he himself was eating. He chose to stop for two weeks to have the conviction and power to make the statement believable to the child. It worked.

This will work for you as you work on yourself. You are the root. Your children are the fruit on the tree. Fix the roots first. Begin by taking one step at a time. It is like eating an elephant. The only way you can possibly do it is one bite at a time. As you begin to live these principles, your life and the lives of your children will be more full and overflowing with the sweet fruit of a healthier and fuller life experience.

Chapter 46
Steps for Healthy Eating

I am a part of all I have met.
—Alfred Lord Tennyson

How do you integrate good habits into your life and the lifestyles of your children? It all begins with attitude.

Food is to be used with an attitude of gratitude. Always have prayer or a moment of meditation before every meal to express gratitude. Eating with an attitude of gratitude is essential. It is hard to express gratitude for the meal you are about to partake of with integrity and then eat something that is harmful to you. Gratitude leads to better habits and greater self-respect.

Learn to treat yourself kindly without the need for food. Do not nurture your emotional self with food. Be kind to yourself in your self-talk. Be forgiving of yourself, as well as others. The better you treat yourself, the less you will need to nurture a wounded self-esteem with food.

Reward good choices and behaviors with expressions of gratitude and appreciation rather than with food. Most parents have observed the effects of simple sugars found in most junk foods and the impact it will have on children's behavior. I have always wondered why parents reward children's good behavior with a treat like candy. After they eat the treat, they act out because of the sugar or other negative ingredients in the food. Their behavior becomes unacceptable, and they get in trouble. The parent just rewarded the child by sabotaging him. We reward them by laying a trap. We reward good behavior by treating them to foods that are "behavioral poison" then punishing them for their undesirable behavior caused by the so-called treat. This is a strange cycle of choice on our part to say the least.

Do not require your children to clean off their plate or to eat all of any specific foods. Some children eat very lightly. As long as they are healthy, don't worry about their sparrow-like eating habits if they are younger than the age of 11.

Eliminate most snack foods, especially just before or after meals. If you do not want the kids eating junk food, don't have it in the house.

Do not be too rigid. Once they enjoy the taste for good food, they will naturally seek to access it more of the time. Do not force them. Give them time, even years. They will gradually follow your lead. Teach them about good nutrition and the reasons for eating well. They will use the knowledge when they are ready to honor it. They will usually honor knowledge as well as you do.

Point out the good feeling that comes from eating good food and the feeling after eating poor-quality food. Children do not know whether the way they feel after eating is normal or not. Ask them. I remember a young girl who on careful questioning revealed that she always had a stomachache after eating. She had never said anything to her mother, because she thought that is what all people experienced. For every meal in her seven years, she had a stomachache. She thought it was normal.

Use food as nutrition, not as a medicine. It is easy to eat well enough to maintain good health. It is more difficult to eat well enough to regain lost vigor and health. Herbs, prescribed according to the principles defined in Chinese medicine, Ayurvedic medicine, or other comprehensive traditions, are a much better way to regain lost balance than trying to eat perfectly.

Eat meals at regular times. It is a marvelous method of growing a unified family and an important part of healthy social development of children. One study demonstrated the more frequently a child ate dinner with his family was the strongest indicator he would be less likely to have problems with drugs, immorality, and lawlessness. In fact, it was the strongest indicator of a "successful" outcome in families.

Eat enough that you are no longer hungry, and then stop. A light diet is one of the main indicators of a long life. If we would reduce our food intake by thirty percent as a society, we would be much healthier. We would also have much more food to share with those less fortunate. Sixty percent of our society is considered overweight. Most of us can afford to eat less.

If a child is very hungry between meals, have him drink more water. Thirst is often misunderstood as hunger. By satisfying our thirst mechanism, we will usually satisfy the real craving that we often perceive as hunger. Water will almost always create good effects in the body. Water should be pure, meaning filtered or distilled. Beverages like fruit juices, soda, or Kool-Aid are not substitutes for water. Water is also best with no ice and close to room temperature. When you drink clean water, it tastes good even at room temperature. Drink to thirst, not out of habit.

You do not have to use all of these steps at one time. Pick one or two that you can integrate without a challenge from the family. Each change you make in this regard will increase your health and the health of your children. As you enjoy greater health in your children, you will experience fewer illnesses. The urgent trips to your pediatrician will be less needed. The need for medication with all the side effects will be lessened if not eliminated. The quality of your life and your child's life will improve. According to my experience, their behavior will become less erratic, more consistent, and more pleasant.

Chapter 47
Fast, Cheap, and Easy Is No Way to Build a Body

It is necessary for the happiness of man that he be
mentally faithful to himself.
—Thomas Paine

Beware the inherent negatives in fast food. The fast foods your children are eating are not of any significant beneficial quality. In fact, they are often made of ingredients, that, if known, no parent would give to his child. Most children who are aware of the ingredients of fast foods do not want to continue eating that type of food. Do some of your own research. Look it up on the Internet. Here are some things for which to look. Which fast food company was the biggest purchaser of Grade "D" chicken meat? Pet food companies do not use less than "C." Which fast food company adds spleen meat to their hamburgers? Which company is the largest purchaser of the thick white "stuff" on the inside of an animals hide before the hide is tanned? They consider it a beef product, do you? Why all the concern over Mad Cow Disease? The current belief is you have to eat the brain and spinal cord to get it. That means some food processors must put those parts in our food, calling it beef; otherwise, there should be little or no concern.

The better your habits are the better your children's habits will be. Always remember, children will mimic the intention behind your activities, not just your choices. Remember the story of Gandhi. Eat right things for the right reasons, and they will get a double dose of goodness. If you don't practice what you preach, neither will they. Pick your message carefully. Make sure you are converted to it. Make sure you will be happy with the outcome. Then do it, and they will follow your lead.

A key to understanding your children is to first know their nature. Honor that. If their behavior is contrary to their nature, you know that something is pushing them in an abnormal direction. Be aware of congruency in their behavior. It will reveal the source of the problem if you tune in to them and carefully observe them. Children, at times, test the limits. We have all done it and seen it. Sometimes they seem irrational in their actions. They may not be testing boundaries; they may be out of control. Seek out the underlying cause and through better nutrition choices help them regain control.

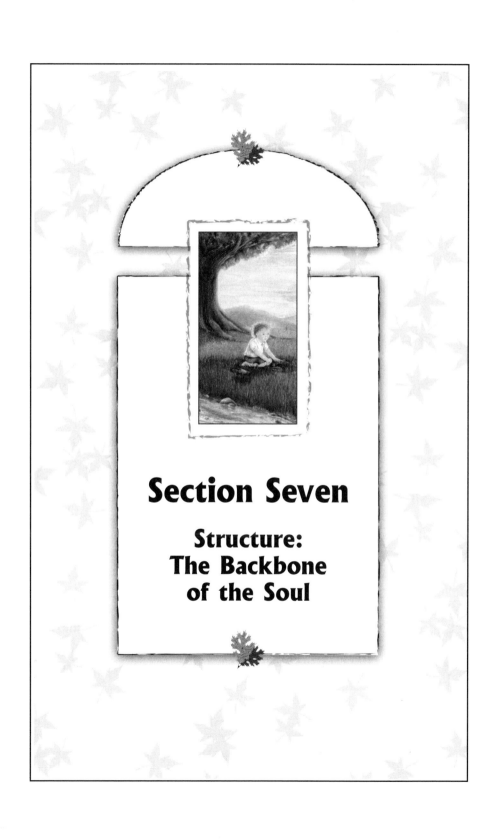

Section Seven

Structure:
The Backbone
of the Soul

Chapter 48
The Nerve System Is in Control

God may forgive your sins, but your nervous system won't.
—Alfred Korzybski

Health is the ability to comprehend yourself in your environment. In the structural or physical body, health is closely integrated to the nerve system. The nerve system communicates all thought into physical reality. Sally sees the ball and decides to kick it; the nerve system transmits that message to the muscles, and thus Sally moves and kicks the ball. Billy decides he is not smart enough to get good grades in school; accordingly, his nerve system will process that thought. Billy believes that thought and, in harmony with it, behaves in a way that will limit his ability to get good grades. Studies have shown that children will achieve their believed potential. It is well documented that you cannot outperform your own self-image. It has also been shown it is difficult to outperform others' image of you. That is why we are the average of the twelve people with whom we spend the most time.

Michelangelo taught from long personal experience, "The greatest danger for most of us is not that our aim is too high and we miss it, but that it is too low and we reach it."

130

In one study, a group of grade school children were tested. The best scoring and worst scoring students were placed in separate groups. The children who scored in the middle were excused. The two groups, the high scoring and low scoring students, were each given a second test. The children who scored poorly on the first test were given unique instructions. They were asked to imagine the smartest person they knew. After they had decided who that was, they were told to imagine they were taking the heads off of their smart friends and putting the smart kids' heads on their bodies. They were asked to take the test with the smart kids' heads on their shoulders. Amazingly, the scores between the two groups, the so-called smart and "dumb kids", were almost identical. The "dumb kids" were told their scores. The researchers commented, "Look how well you did." The kids responded, "It was Bobby or Suzy that made that score. I couldn't do that." The way we think, good or bad, is transmitted to the body through the nervous system. Therefore, the thinking we create is transmitted into physical reality through this process.

Chapter 49
Spinal Alignment Is the Keystone to Structural Health

*Spine transplants are what we really need
to take Reagan on.*
—Pat Schroeder

Health is built on communication. Communication between our body, mind, and spirit is critical. Fundamental to this is the communication between different systems in our body. Each part of the body needs to be able to freely and accurately communicate with every other part. The major communication system in the body is the brain and nervous system. The brain gives instructions to every part of our body through the nervous system; the body responds and sends messages back. The accuracy of those instructions and the precision with which they are carried out determines to a large degree our level of health physically, emotionally, and spiritually.

As the brain receives a message or stimulus, it categorizes the message. It will then choose to ignore the message or to respond. The response is sent to the body as a series of messages that come as reactions. If the stomach sends a message to the brain that it is full, the brain will send a message to the rest of the body that it is time to stop eating. If that message is not received accurately, the person may continue to eat. Anything that creates interference in any nervous system message will cause disharmony. This disharmony causes abnormal function, which leads to physical distress. This physical breakdown in communication will lead to lack of health and probable symptoms. Such a condition may result in serious consequences or perhaps just annoying symptoms that lessen our quality of life. If we treat the symptom and ignore the underlying cause, nerve interference, if it is present, we are not improving long-term quality of life or caring for health.

The spine is critical to good health. One of the main functions of the spine is to protect the nervous system. The brain by means of the nervous system controls the body. Any interference in the normal nervous system function will create a problem in the body. The spine is the great protector of the spinal cord and the spinal nerves that control every part of the body.

If the spine is traumatized, it often goes out of its ideal alignment. When this very common condition happens, it causes interference in the nervous system's ability to regulate the body. Nerve interference is, in my experience, a major contributor to poor health in our society.

Chapter 50
The Missing Expert

All of us are experts at practicing virtue at a distance.
—Theodore Hesburg

The most highly trained experts in our society who find and eliminate nerve interference are doctors of chiropractic. When there is nerve interference in our bodies, we will not enjoy optimal health. Medical doctors are experts in disease. Chiropractors are experts in health. Chiropractors are the masters at finding and correcting nerve interference in the spine, called a subluxation. A subluxation is when a vertebra "goes out" of its proper alignment. This misalignment of a vertebra always causes nerve interference. A specific chiropractic adjustment is the best way of removing subluxations and the associated nerve interference.

Even though subluxations always cause nerve interference, they do not always cause pain. Only a small portion of the nerves that passes out of the spine to the body have to do with pain sensations. Even without pain, subluxations always cause some level of "dis-ease." I have seen specific chiropractic adjustments remove nerve interference, allowing the body's self-healing mechanisms to correct such conditions as otitis media, asthma, constipation, pain, headaches, nausea, jaw pain, poor digestion, crossed eyes, sinus problems, bed wetting, premenstrual syndrome, and many other conditions. But the most stunning thing I have seen chiropractors improve is health, vibrancy in life, increased energy, increased happiness, less stressful life, and a life more full of joy. It is important to note that chiropractic is a method of treating cause, not symptoms. By removing nerve interference, the underlying cause of "dis-ease" is addressed. This allows the body's normal, God-given, healing mechanisms to operate. Health returns as soon as the body's self-contained, healing mechanism can get the job done. When more of the areas of SENSE, structural in this case, are balanced, healing will happen more quickly and more completely.

We generally get our teeth checked twice a year. We have our cholesterol and our blood pressure checked. We take our children to a pediatrician to have them screened for early onset of disease. Why not get the most important system in the body tuned up on a regular basis? You get your car serviced, change the oil in your lawn mower, and get your eyes checked. Getting a regular, spinal checkup is critical to well-being, because nerve interference can be silent and serious. Subluxations cause vital information to be distorted, and not having them removed can have serious, long-term health consequences.

Chapter 51
Caring for the Cause

Life is a perpetual instruction in cause and effect.
—Ralph Waldo Emerson

One day a mother brought in her son for care. He was sixteen months old and had a severe case of constipation. Every day of his life he had felt the pressure and pain of abnormal bowel function. She had tried every medical option, some very unpleasant, to no avail. He continued to have the problem and the associated struggles whenever the pressure of elimination occurred. I gave him a thorough examination and found only one likely cause of his problem. He had a subluxated vertebra in the lowest section of his spine down by his tailbone. This is the area where the nerves that control the bowels are located. This subluxation was causing nerve interference on the very nerves that controlled the lower bowels. I talked to the mother and explained this to her. I delivered a precise adjustment to the vertebrae that was subluxated. As usual, it caused no distress to the boy. Two days later, when the mother brought him back, she reported that he had had his first normal bowel movement ever. We adjusted him again, and his problem resolved and never returned. It seemed that he had nerve messages blocked in the lower bowel area that led to this abnormal, bowel function. Removal of the nerve interference by gentle chiropractic adjustments removed the cause and allowed the body to express its normal level of health. He then returned to get regular, chiropractic care to keep his spine healthy and free of nerve interference.

What would have been the consequences of this subluxation in forty years time if he had not been adjusted? He could have had almost any type of bowel condition or disease develop and had the pain and discomfort from this condition for the rest of his life. Two simple adjustments removed the nerve interference that was the underlying cause of his problem. Free flow of nerve energy returned, and his body was able to comprehend itself in its environment; health returned, and normal nerve and bowel function became standard. No other treatment would have ever removed the underlying cause, and no other treatment would have removed the cause of the constipation while improving his general well-being. When there is nerve interference present, no other adaptation will work to correct the cause of the problem. Medication may provide temporary relief but will not remedy the cause. The nerve interference must be removed.

Chapter 52
Living Proof of the Supremacy of the Spine

Cab drivers are living proof that
practice does not make perfect.
—Howard Ogden

Masha and Dasha were identical twins, joined at the waist. They had four arms, but just two legs. They shared every system in the body but the central nervous system, meaning the brain and spinal cord. The blood that flowed in one flowed in the other. They shared digestive function and even respiratory function. Amazingly, as they grew, one of them would catch a cold, but the other one did not; yet, they shared the same blood. How could one have a cold, and the same blood containing the virus circulated in the other twin, yet she did not catch the cold? The only system that was unique to each girl was the nervous system. One could have subluxations, and the other would not. Individual thought had independent effect on each girl. Thus, one could get sick and the other stay healthy, because she had healthy nervous system function, meaning no subluxations.

A body is only as healthy as the spine. They were proof that nerve interference will compromise the immune system and every other system in the body, whereas a healthy spine and nervous system will keep every other system in the body finely tuned. You could look at a picture of Masha and Dasha and guess which one got sick. The posture of the sick twin was not as good as her sisters. The better posture proved a healthier child.

In my family, I have seen the effects of spinal adjustments. My children have never really been sick. I believe their wellness has been attributable to good spinal health, along with other healthy habits. As mentioned previously, each area of SENSE has a deep effect on overall health. If any one of the areas is out of balance, it can compromise the overall health of a child.

Chapter 53
The Most Important Checkup Your Child Can Have

As the twig is bent, so grows the tree.
—German proverb

Have you had your child's spine checked for subluxations? If you have not, you have missed one of the easiest and most critical aspects to sustaining and maintaining great health. As you keep your children subluxation-free you will observe a marked improvement in their health and happiness. Nobody can be as healthy with nerve interference as without. For your child to truly reach his amazing promise, a free functioning nervous system is an absolute necessity. Some of you will see miracles when you have your child cared for by a nervous system expert, a chiropractor. Keep getting their teeth checked every six months but have their spine checked at least every month, a small investment to grasp the full measure of promise God placed in your child.

140

Chapter 54
Posture: The Reflection of Inner Dynamics

The doctor of the future will give not medicine but will inter-est his patient in the care of the human frame, in diet and the cause and prevention of disease.
—Thomas Edison

Erect posture is vital to good spinal health and free nerve system expression. Great posture is made up of a subluxation-free spine, good muscle balance, and emotional balance. Posture is affected by personality characteristics, genetic tendencies, habits, and what we learn from our mentors. We know from deep experience that our emotions affect our posture, and our posture affects our emotions. I believe that our emotions make a more important contribution to our posture than any other factor outside of spinal subluxations. If we feel good about ourselves, our posture will tend to be more erect. We will look others directly in the eye, our shoulders will be held back in an erect posture, and our head will be held high. Why does the military teach soldiers to have an erect posture? It makes them feel more confident, more powerful, and invincible. It also makes them stronger with better endurance. When we help our children feel confident, powerful, and invincible, they will stand erect, look people in the eye, and speak clearly with a confident voice. In accordance with the entire premise of this book, if you want your children to have good posture, teach them to feel good about themselves. Help them see themselves as they really are. As they catch the vision of their true potential, they will stand tall in any situation. Be aware of your own posture. Harping on them about their posture is the least effective way to change their postural habits. Find their virtue and convince them of it. Convince yourself of it. When you believe they are unique and special, they will begin to believe, also. When you see their true nature and recognize their gifts, you will know they are special and treat them accordingly. When you know they are unique and special, they will believe it. As soon as you believe they are special, they will have the power to act out of their amazing, authentic selves. They will lose the need to please others. They will not need to respond to others' attitudes and words. They will act out of their own, inner integrity and allow others the same right. They will become a stable influence in life and in your family. They will begin to stand tall and erect-structurally, morally, emotionally, and mentally.

Chapter 55
Structural Integrity a Step at a Time

One step at a time is good walking.
—Chinese proverb

What are your children's strength? Be creative. Be thoughtful.

_____

_____

_____

What do you wish their strength were? Be honest. Who needs to change here, you or them?

_____

_____

_____

If you extend their strengths, what does that mean your children can become?

_____

_____

_____

How can you help them use those strengths to their advantage?

_____

_____

_____

When you believe in their strengths, what impact do you believe you will see in their behavior?

_____

_____

_____

Chapter 56
Your Children Are True to Themselves

This is the true joy in life - being used for a purpose recognized by yourself as a mighty one.
—George Bernard Shaw

It is impossible to celebrate your children's strengths and be critical of them. Children will always be true to the view they have of themselves. I repeat; children will always be true to the view they have of themselves. If you do not like their behavior, first understand the way you see them and the way they view themselves. Recognize they are usually playing a role. They believe they are supposed to be that way. Help them see themselves as they really are with all of their virtues. There is not a child who is not full and overflowing with virtue. Once you see them as extraordinary, they will begin to believe it; and when they see themselves as they really are, they will be able to look at life as it really is. They will not accept responsibility for others' happiness and not need others to be happy for them to be happy. They will then be free to make their own choices and do so with appropriate awareness. They will be able to act in their environment in a free and easy manner. They will learn to act rather than react and will gain the ability to be rather than just do.

145

Chapter 57
See Them as They Can Be

Allow children to be happy in their own way,
for what better way will they find?
—Samuel Johnson

Picture your children in your mind's eye in their goodness and incredible, divine nature. How would they stand if they could see themselves in this way? Close your eyes, and picture them. See them as God sees them. Imagine them being fully aware of themselves and their true potential. Visualize them being able to act out of their virtue rather than reacting to others. See them being fully confident in themselves in all situations. Do you want this possibility for your children? If we can see them as they really are and treat them with that image in our hearts, you will give them that possibility. They then have the power to use their God-given right to choose, their moral agency, to take advantage of this gift. We must give them that right. If we attempt to suppress their divinely appointed privilege, they will struggle against us mightily. In all situations, children have the power to choose their responses. Wisely used, this power expands to a creativity that can magically turn any situation into an opportunity.

When my oldest daughter was about ten years old, there was a young boy who took a liking to her. He became a very persistent suitor. He would call her nearly every day. She never wanted to talk to him. She tried to communicate to him that she was not interested in him or in having a boyfriend, but he kept calling. I started talking to him more when he would call. One day, as I was chatting with him I told him, "You certainly can talk."

He responded with, "My teacher told me I have a big mouth."

"Really," I responded a little surprised that a teacher would say something like that. "Did that bother you that your teacher told you that?" I asked him.

"No, I took it as a compliment. Why would I want to be offended? I just took it as a compliment. It meant to me that I can talk well, and I like to talk. I wasn't offended," he replied. What a great choice! Look at the power that choice had on that boy. That teacher's statement could have damaged his self-opinion if he had chosen to take it in a different way. He could have become shy, withdrawn, and self-conscious. Instead he chose to take it as a compliment. You cannot offend someone without his permission. He retained the right to not be offended. He made a wise choice, and he was right; he was a good talker. That was real. He did not have a big mouth; it was the same size as every other child's mouth. He was not concerned with what the teacher thought of him. He was only concerned with what he felt about himself. What someone else thought about him was that person's choice and problem, and he preserved the incredible power of good self-image.

Chapter 58
Laugh or Cry

When a father gives to his son, both laugh;
when a son gives to his father, both cry.
—William Shakespeare

I remember sitting in front of a grocery store one day in my car as my wife ran in for a quick purchase. As I sat there, a man walked out of the store with a small sack. He had a unique and bizarre posture and gait. He walked somewhat like a chicken. He leaned way forward, moving his head back and forth with each step in a dramatic, chicken-like fashion. I almost chuckled at the unique walk. Suddenly, I noticed a young man who worked at the store walking out behind this man, mimicking him in an over-exaggeration of the unique "chicken" walk.

This time I did laugh. Then, I felt for the man. If he turned around and saw the clown-like parody being played out behind him, he could certainly be offended and perhaps have hurt feelings. Suddenly, it dawned on me that the young man was not fooling around. He was the man's son. His father was picking him up after work. He had learned to walk like his father, only in an exaggeration of the father's quirks of kinesthesia. Wow!

Be a Positive Example

We teach our children so many powerful lessons! If the father had set out to make his son walk like him, he could not have done it, but by being a silent example, which the son chose to emulate, the son became an exaggeration of his father's pattern of being, right down to his posture. With that posture, he also undoubtedly learned to assimilate the feelings and emotions that accompany that physical form and movement. He may even have integrated certain physical flaws into his life that the father had as well. What a powerful example we are to our children.

Build Rich Soil

It is believed that up to eighty percent of communication is through body language. As parents, we create the soil that our children, who are really seeds of divinity, are planted in. We get to create the soil from which they grow. As much as the potential of the seed, the nature of the soil determines the sweetness of the fruit. Create it mindfully. The sweetness of our golden years is grown out of such well-tended soil.

We Are Amazing Teachers

We need to learn to be aware of our teaching. Most of it is subconscious and unintended. We teach much more by what we are than by what we say or even what we yell. Our actions are always much louder than our words. We teach the strongest lessons out of the integrity of our being. That which we are is communicated loudly to all around us, especially our children. How many of you have caught yourself doing or saying something that your parents used to do or say that you promised you would never do, and later in life you become exactly what you promised you would never be. These lessons are powerful and revealing of our internal integrity. Our children will be like us in intricate ways that we would be wise to recognize. Sometimes this mimicking creates the very disdain some children express toward their parents. By mimicking the parents, they create inner conflict, because they are different than their parents. We all know that some children have different personalities than the parents from the beginning. Yet, we usually want them to fall in line and walk like a duck, even if they have fur and four legs. Allow the child to have his own personality, and he will accept you as you accept him, despite the inherent differences. Celebrate his strengths. Find his virtue, and trumpet it. To vocalize his lack or to harp on his weaknesses only drives a wedge between what he knows of himself and what you seem to believe of him. The first thing to fail is his belief in you. The second is his belief in himself. We are powerful role models.

Chapter 59
Maybe You Can Help My Son!

My childhood should have taught me lessons for my
fatherhood, but it didn't because parenting can only be
learned by people who have no children.
—Bill Cosby

I knew a massage therapist who specialized in Rolfing, a deep method of muscle work, and had the following experience. He treated a man one day who had fallen off a barn roof six years earlier. He had broken his pelvis, leg, and ankle. The injury caused a marked limp and lingering gait abnormality. He swiveled his hips and swung one leg in a strange and unorthodox manner with each labored step. After the first session of Rolfing, the man was so pleased with the improvement that he told the massage therapist, "If you helped me, I am sure you would be able to help my son." "What is the matter with your son," asked the massage therapist. "I will go get him. He is out in the car," he replied. In a moment the man came in with his six-year-old son walking beside him. The boy walked just like his father. He had the same, unique walk, but he had never fallen off a barn roof. He had never broken his pelvis, leg, or ankle. He had observed his father and mimicked him so well he walked in the same way. As the massage therapist worked on the boy, he noted the same, unusual, tight muscles and compensations as he had seen in the father. The boy had never fallen off the barn roof; yet he carried the effects of the trauma in a deep, physical way like his father did.

Do Your Best

Recognize what a powerful force you are in your child's life. We can be a solid force for good, or we can be a devastating force that brings pain and challenge. If you are consistent, your children will gradually learn to use the force of your mistakes for good, just like a sailor can use almost any wind to sail toward his objective. Do not expect to be perfect; just be your best. Children, above all else, are forgiving. Do your best; be consistent and loving. With that beginning they will raise us into loving adults who can give more to the world than we ever thought possible. I do believe that children teach parents far more than parents need to teach children. If we love them, they will learn all they need. If we seek to teach them, we usually end up manipulating them to the detriment of all involved. If we were truly supposed to be the best possible teachers of children, God would send children to the wisest and most loving of us all. He would not let humans have children until they reached the age of wisdom and maturity. So children come to this life to help raise parents, at least in part.

As we honor this role, we will help teach our children to be their best. When they are at their best, they will express it in their posture.

Chapter 60
The Critical Ingredients to Postural Integrity

*The strength of a nation derives from
the integrity of the home.*
—Confucius

• Be the best example you can be of good posture and moral integrity.

• Find the child's virtue and celebrate it. The question is not, "How good is my child?" but, "How is my child good?" Make a list.

• Help your child convince himself of his goodness.

• Improve postural alignment by removing nerve inter-ference caused by subluxations.

• Create exercise habits. Instill some physical activity, not necessarily sport. John Gray, author of *Men Are from Mars and Women Are from Venus*, has stated that thirty minutes of exercise every day with a B-complex supplement has shown to be seven times more effective than Ritalin at treating ADHD.

- Let babies lie on the floor. Allow them to learn to lift their heads and then get on their knees. Let them learn to crawl. This is critical for the development of spinal health and flexibility.

- Avoid walkers and baby swings. My experience teaches me that these implements cause many structural, postural, and nervous system problems that will linger through their lives, a high price to pay for apparent momentary advantage.

- Teach them to walk when they are ready. They will learn in their time.

- Stimulate your child's sensory energy system by gentle massage.

- Participate with your children in physical activities. Balance mind play, like video games, with an equal amount of physical activity.

- Get your child and yourself checked out by a highly referred chiropractor.

- Get their spine checked and aligned monthly.

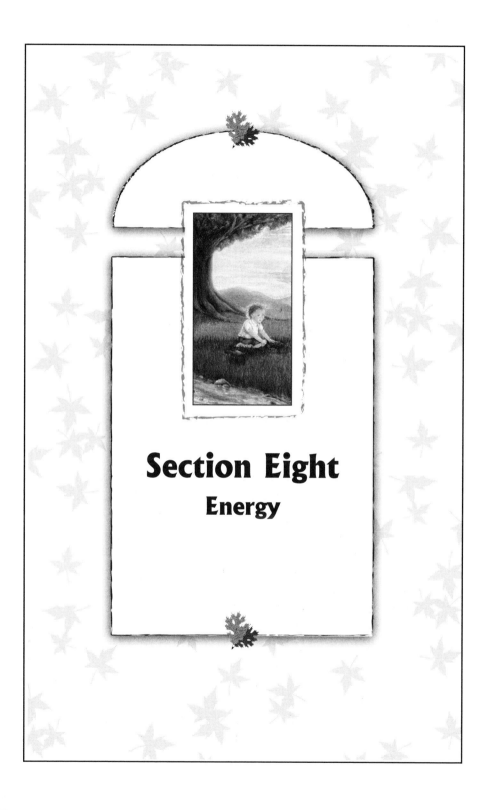

Section Eight
Energy

Chapter 61
You Have More Energy
Than You Thought

Love is an energy which exists of itself. It is its own value.
—Thornton Wilder

Energy is a term that is vague and at the same time extraordinarily specific. To achieve and maintain a balance of energy is a stabilizing factor in every other aspect of SENSE. In the West, the term energy is used very broadly and generally. Maybe you have heard someone say, "I don't have enough energy." Or, "She has good energy." "He has bad energy." And maybe you have expressed, "Wow, they are an energy drainer." Yet, there is little definition given to this term "energy."

To understand energy a little better, let's consider that a culture is made up of people. People are made up of systems that are made of organs. Organs are made of tissues, which are made of cells, which are made and constructed of subcellular organisms, which are made of molecules. Molecules are made of atoms, which are built of subatomic particles, which are made of...energy. In the end, when we look at all matter, it is made of energy. The study of energy on this level is called quantum physics. This is the level of science that Einstein and his peers chose to study to better understand the universe in which we live. Everything is energy.

Yet, we do not think of it that way. We see the world around us as being substantial and solid. The substance of the world we know, matter, is really more like a scene out of a science fiction movie than the way we perceive it. Let me use an illustration. Hydrogen, the smallest atom, is made of one nucleus and one electron. If we could increase its scale so its size is equal to that of a large college football stadium, the nucleus would be only the size of a grain of salt, and the electron would be much smaller than that. The hydrogen atom is almost all space.

The same is basically true of all atoms. They are 99.999% space, with the nucleus and electrons as dancing specks of energy. The "inner space" of matter, meaning the atomic or quantum level of things, is made up of similar proportions as outer space. When we travel to space, the planets seem so far apart. Yet, in inner space the relationships of size and space are similar. It is easy to travel in outer space without running into some other object. Inner space is just as vast and wide open. Keep in mind that we are really energetic beings, even if we feel we are solid and firm.

Chapter 62
Like Children, Energy Is
Always Moving

If we continually try to force a child to do what he is afraid
to do, he will become more timid, and will use his brains
and energy, not to explore the unknown, but to find ways to
avoid the pressure we put on him.
—John R. Holt, Jr.

The Chinese system of healing has identified energy channels in the body. These energy channels are the main conduits of energy movement in the body. Energy, like us, cannot stand still. We may be able to be idle or stationary, but we cannot truly stand still. Movement of our blood, nerve energy, tissue development or breakdown is always present. We are like an ant pile of movement. This is true of energy channels, also. These channels are separated into fourteen main energy pathways. The energy flows in a predictable manner, direction, and time-related pattern. Every day at specific times the life energy, or qi' (pronounced chi'), moves into different areas of emphasis. At 2 AM, it is in the liver area, at 6 AM, it is in the large intestine area. Proper balance of the energy in the body channels is a vital predictor of health. This is the focus of acupuncture and Chinese herbology, as well as some types of bodywork like massage therapy and shiatsu. For three thousand years, the Chinese and other Eastern cultures have been using, developing, and proving the efficacy of this system.

Many systems of exercise and thought are designed around energy balance. Taiji, yoga, qigong, and meditation systems are based on achieving energy balance. Energy balance is a vital aspect of health. The good news is you do not have to do any or all of these practices to find energetic balance.

Chapter 63
Energy Is the By-product of Our Choices

When you make a choice you activate vast human energies
and resources that otherwise go untapped.
—Robert Fritz

In Chinese theory, the statement, "The Yi (mind) leads the qi (energy or life force)," implies the reality that the mind is the controller of the energy. The way we think in reality changes the way the energy circulates in the body. The movement and flow of energy will affect the body chemistry and tissue integrity. What is the mind other than a tool of choice? We receive data, "Suzy screams." We analyze the data. "That is just how Suzy always screams when Billy punches her." We make deductions and decisions (or choices) from that data. "Billy must have punched Suzy again." Then we act based on the choice we have made. "Bill, go to your room for the next hour." After the choice has been turned into action, consequences arise. Suzy sits triumphantly on the pile of toys she has pilfered from Billy and grins at how easy it was to manipulate the system. Energy arises out of the thought, emotion, and the action. Suzy is enjoying the temporary high of a corporate raider, whereas Billy is frustrated and feels misunderstood and cheated. Energy may seem similar to emotion. It is a by-product of our emotional states. Emotion is the result of our spiritual perspective and our life circumstances. Energy is the by-product of our choices. These choices are the product of our spiritual nature, circumstances, and attitudes.

Energy Is Choice

Energy is actually just that, energy, but it is controlled and created in us by choice. In the book of Genesis, God told Adam and Eve not to eat of the forbidden fruit. Then He followed with the essential council, "Nevertheless thou mayest choose for thyself." In this God gave Adam and Eve power to choose and the ability to receive consequences for action and choice. That choice is creative is beyond question. Each choice we make has consequences. There are laws set before the foundations of the world that have built-in consequences. Our interaction with the divine is on God's terms, not on our own. We can choose our actions; however, we cannot choose the consequences of our actions. We must choose our life based on long-term consequences and integrity to who we really are.

In our interaction with other people, we cannot know whether the data we receive is complete or not. We may experience something, but the fact that we do not gather all of the critical information that went into that event is undeniable. We cannot know if we are making completely correct or accurate decisions based on the data we receive. As a result, we make the best decision we can on the basis of our perception. The more our perception is based on reality, the greater the likelihood we experience joy in this life. The inherent effects of decisions, good or bad, bring lessons that teach the virtue lacking in the circumstance. Next time such a situation arises we will be more able to choose wisely. The very effect of our decision is the creation of energy.

Chapter 64
Dynamo or Dynamite

*I cannot conceive a rank more honorable, than that which
flows from the uncorrupted choice of a brave and free
people, the purest source and original fountain of all power.*
—George Washington

Let's use a hypothetical situation. Imagine for me, with the incredible creative mind you have, that you have just had an amazingly challenging day. You have had three flat tires and two tow truck rides. You dropped your groceries leaving the grocery store, and ruined almost everything. In addition, you gave away the winning lottery ticket for sixty million dollars before you knew it was a winner, and your spouse lost his job. Both children got sent to the principal's office, and the principal is now on your case. Yuck! You finally make it home at the end of the day. You close the door behind you, and you lean against it. No more today thank goodness, you think. Just then, the phone rings. Your first impulse is to let it ring. You are afraid if you answer it you might wring it like a wet washcloth. Your better senses prevail; you make a choice, and pick up the phone, "Hello?" It is your best friend, who sounds panicked. "My youngest child was

just killed in a hit-and-run car accident. Can you come help me?
I can't handle this."

What is your response? I am sure you would instantly weigh
your bad day, compare it quickly to hers, and say, "I will be right
there!" Your fatigue, frustration, depression, and/or irritation
disappear. In an instant you transform yourself from an emotional and physical wreck to an energized dynamo capable of
anything to help your friend in this time of great need. You did it
instantly and by simply making a choice. The power of one
choice is immense. You could have made the choice to rid yourself of those negative mindsets without your friend needing to
lose a child. But by making a choice you change from being set
on by life to being a savior for your friend. By recognition of
choice you learn to access the higher levels of choice. Therein lies
true power. Sometimes we need extreme situations to empower
us, but the power lies in our choice. Choice is the true instigator
of energy.

Chapter 65
Energy Controls Our Body

Today is yesterday's effect and tomorrow's cause.
—Phillip Gribble

What are the physical effects of this choice? Are your shoulders as tight? Is your blood pressure as high? What brain chemicals changed in your body with that decision? Do you feel more energized? Is your mood the same? Does serotonin change levels? What about dopamine? Is your energy different? All these factors change with the choice to drop your current, believed, emotional woes and help your friend. It all changed because of a small choice. In fact, most of this choice is subconscious. You did not evaluate every aspect of this decision. You made it based on your inner virtue. If we look at reality, the moment before the phone rang, the child was still dead, your friend was still distraught, and your day was what you thought it was, or was it? You were leaning against the wall, and you were centered on your own self-created woes. Were they real? In one sense they were. But a moment after answering the phone and making a different choice, how real were they now? Was your day really so bad? Apparently, it was not. What power a choice has! How did you

164

manage to change your state of mind? You let go of your self-pity to grab hold of a higher virtue of empathy, and you acted out of that higher virtue.

So, the quality of our virtue determines the quality of our energy. I am not talking about just vim and vigor. By energy, I mean the resource that your body is made of and can access to create. Virtue lies in the purity of the motivation, not in our proclaimed intention.

Chapter 66
Love Is Pure Energy

Love the moment and the energy of the moment will
spread beyond all boundaries.
—Corita Kent

Love, in the pure SENSE, does not require an outcome. In the common use of the word love, we need those around us to behave the way we want them to. When we do something nice, we want a specific response, and if we do not get it, we are upset. Thus, our motive was to get the reaction we desired. When we can do some noble thing for another and not need a reaction, we are getting closer to love. The higher quality virtues are made of pure and virtuous motives. The consequences of choices are not cut and dried, but they are consistent. Circumstances will create different effects even with the same action. For example, jumping always has the effect that you will come down. Jumping off the ground will have the reaction of coming down on the ground. Jumping off a tall building will have a different reaction. You will come down, but the effect of that reaction will be in accordance with the other factors at work.

Again, the effect of jumping off a building will be very different if you have attached yourself to a hang glider, and the effect will vary again if you know how to use the hang glider. If there is a strong wind, the effect will be different than the other scenarios.

Understanding energy is to understand the effects of actions in the system in which you are. Much of the reason we are on this earth is to learn this singular lesson. If you knew the effects of your actions in totality before you undertook them, you would have an entirely different manner of acting. By cultivating the ability to know the consequence of your actions, you create an energetic awareness.

Deeper insight to ponder: Energy is the second subtlest field of awareness next to spirit. Awareness of energy gives awareness of intent, both yours and others' at a physical or emotional level, but not at a spiritual level. A person very tuned into energy can give you information and insight at an energetic or emotional level of reality, but not in the realm of things spiritual. Often in our society, we have intermingled the energetic and spiritual realms, but they are separate and very distinct. Energetic awareness is not directly connected to spiritual realities. Just because someone is psychic, he is not necessarily prophetic. Spiritual realities are a level that energetic awareness cannot discriminate. Things of a spiritual nature must be viewed on a separate plane. Just as there are different levels of physical laws, so is there with spiritual laws. All levels of spiritual laws have reality, but only the highest levels can see the lower levels in totality. Be careful not to confuse energetic awareness with a spiritual awareness.

Chapter 67
Energy Is Choice

Power is the vital energy to make choices and decisions.
—Anonymous

We have the God-given right to choose. We get to act as an individual with given and set physical, energetic, and spiritual consequences to our actions. We can act, or we can be acted on by life's circumstances, but if we use our right to choose wisely, we will always retain the right to act and not just react. If you choose to break the law, you will lose the right to go on a picnic with your family when you want because you will probably be in jail. By expressing your freedom to drink and drive drunk, you will eventually lose rights. By choosing wisely our choices remain open. If your boss comes in one day and chews you out for no reason and you remain calm, allowing him the right to be angry and let it pass, you preserve the right to continue to work there or to quit and go work someplace else. If you loose your cool and fight back against your perceptions, you may lose your job and the right to choose your path in that thing. This is the reason for God's counsel to us that we call commandments. The commandments are not a limiting guideline but a command to stay free to choose. As long as we choose wisely, we can retain the right to continue choosing. If we choose unwisely, we narrow our choices. Such is it with our children. One wise man said that you could tell your children no longer need guidance when they stop resenting it.

Chapter 68
Act and Stay Free

Mankind's greatest gift, also its greatest curse,
is that we have free choice.
—Elisabeth Kubler-Ross

Teach your children to act and not react. All practices that cultivate an awareness of energy will heighten our perception of the ability to choose. If one develops the practice of an energetic martial art like taiji (a gentle martial art that focuses on awareness and sensitivity), one will be able, in circumstances that may limit some people's choices, to retain the right to choose a response and to act out of ability rather than out of negative emotion. If a bully challenges, one will be able to choose personal action when others will more than likely choose to react. In reacting, the platform of choice is a negative emotion, virtue, or circumstance. A truly positive outcome from a negative platform is hard to imagine. When we reserve the right to act, we retain the ability to be positive, virtuous, and loving. When we react, we are acting on the foundation of the original act performed by the other person. Thus, we are out of our own control and under his control. I believe that others can only influence us at the level and to the degree we give them power over us. Thus we are judging and falling into the trap of acting with insufficient information.

Aikido is a martial art that focuses on being centered and aware of the peaceful path in life and the recognition that outer conflict is only a manifestation of inner conflict. One young man went to Japan to study aikido and further his considerable skill with the martial art. After two years of full-time study in Japan, he was returning home on the late train after a day of hard training. At one stop, a large Japanese man got on the train. He was drunk and seemed angry. He caused quite a commotion. The aikido practitioner observed him but remained calm and uninvolved. The drunken man was aggressive and abusive, both verbally and physically, to those around him. When he shoved down a pregnant lady and started trying to tear out a pole on the train, the kind that passengers use to hold onto, the aikido practitioner decided it was time to put a stop to this potentially dangerous situation. He learned in aikido not to be confrontational, but he saw no way around this situation. As he drew near the drunken man, he was noticed. They exchanged words. Just as a physical encounter became almost inevitable and all the other people on the train had scattered, a small, thin, reedy voice behind the drunk man called out, "Hey you! Have you been drinking?" The drunken man turned and responded, "Yeah, what's it to you?"

"Have you been drinking sake?"

"Yeah, so what?"

"I love to drink sake," said an old withered Japanese man. "In the evening like this when I get home late, my wife has a warm pot of sake. We go out back in my beautiful rock garden and we sit and we drink sake by the light of the stars. It is so beautiful. I love to be with my wife. It is my favorite time of the day. Do you have a wife?" The large man slumped, his shoulders sagging and replied, "My wife left me. Now I have lost my job. That's why I was drinking." The old man was compassionate, "Oh, I am sorry. Come over here. Come sit by me. Do you love your wife?" asked the old man.

"Yes, she meant everything to me," replied the large drunk.

Before long the drunk was lying on the bench next to the old man, who held his head in his lap as the large man wept and talked about the challenges he was facing, with his wife leaving him and then losing his job and the fears of loneliness and the unknown that had overtaken him.

The aikido practitioner saw the pain that could be caused in the situation; the old man saw a soul in pain. The aikido practitioner saw with his eyes; the old man saw with his heart. The young man would have added insult to a tender soul and a broken heart. The old man touched a life, a heart, and a soul in a gentle loving way. The aikido practitioner reacted. The old man acted. The young man would have lost his genuine power. The old man expanded his power and that of everyone present.

Those who act develop the ability to inspire. Those who react can only conspire. Those who cultivate the virtue of pure love have the greatest ability of any to "act" in all circumstances. They never have a need to react. They who act out of love have the greatest energetic balance. Perfect love brings perfect harmony and perfect energetic balance. Perfect balance brings perfect health. Perfect health brings the ability to experience life fully. Perfect health is not necessarily a life without any physical challenge; it is a life of full awareness of the wonders in the universe.

Chapter 69
Seek the Highest in You

*The end of wisdom is to dream high enough to lose
the dream in the seeking for it.*
—William Faulkner

To seek the highest energetic balance requires that we also seek balance in all other areas of health, or SENSE. To find and attain balance requires us to seek to find the path that is made of love in its highest and finest aspects. One man demonstrated this principle in a powerful story.

During World War II there were terrible examples of man's inhumanity to man. After the war was over and the concentration camps were opened, there was much hatred among the weak and emaciated survivors. In one camp observers noticed a native of Poland who seemed so robust and peaceful they thought he must have only recently been imprisoned. They were surprised to learn that he had been there over six years! Then, they reasoned, he must not have suffered the terrible atrocities to his family members that most of the prisoners had. But in questioning him, they learned how soldiers had come to his city, lined up against a wall his wife, two daughters, and three small sons, then opened fire with a machine gun. Though he begged to die with them, he had been kept alive because of his knowledge and ability in language translation.

This Polish father said: "I had to decide right then...whether to let myself hate the soldiers who had done this. It was an easy decision, really. I was a lawyer. In my practice I had seen...what hate could do to people's minds and bodies. Hate had just killed the six people who mattered most to me in the world. I decided then that I would spend the rest of my life-whether it was a few days or many years-loving every person I came in contact with" (George G. Ritchie with Elizabeth Sherrill, Return from Tomorrow, Waco, Texas: Chosen Books, 1978, p. 116).

Energy Is Choice

One choice made and honored can have incredible power in life. What a powerful change choice can make in the world. Choose to follow at least one of the simple steps at the end of each section. Select one activity that you are not currently doing in your family. Be diligent and persistent, and watch the changes that take place in your life and the lives of your children. Continue to add another step as you feel ready. Keep it up until you are practicing all the steps that fit into your life. You will be amazed at the change in your outlook and the outlook of your family members. Your life will expand in power, freedom, peace, happiness, and love. The essence of health is power. The result of true power is joy. May you seek and find the joy of powerfully directed choice in your life.

Chapter 70
Steps to Help Teach Choice

Give to every child a good example, to yourself, respect.
—Anonymous

• Your example: Be ever mindful of your choices and what you communicate to others as you act out of conscious choice.

• Teach your children situation by situation that they have the right to choose.

• Teach them that no one else can dictate their feelings.

• They are good no matter what happens. Acts do not equal value. Always treat the child as a virtuous person. Criticism is unhelpful in any situation.

• Every circumstance creates choice and thus potential. Celebrate every situation that brings choice.

• Prayer, meditation, yoga, taiji, qigong, or other practices can help teach inner awareness and the power of choice. Investigate one of them as a possible practice to clarify your life.

- Ask your children questions. Encourage them to ask questions. Be patient in answering their questions. They are great question askers. Teach them self-awareness by asking them good questions about why they made their choices.

- Cultivate talents. This broadens our choices. Help each member of your family choose one new talent to enhance. What do they really wish they could do? Help them work toward accomplishing that thing.

- Treat your children as your special assignment from God. Christ taught that of "such is the kingdom of heaven." In reality they are closer to God in character and attribute than you are.

- By honoring your children, you honor yourself. You are also magnificent. Believe you are, and you can believe your children are.

Epilogue

Man is greater than the world - than a system of worlds;
there is more mystery in the union of soul with the body
than in the creation of a universe.
—Henry Giles

Life is made up of choices. The universe is abundant with unlimited opportunities. You have an opportunity now to choose where you are going to live among the endless levels of realities that you can choose and create. Are you going to choose to stay the same, or are you going to choose the challenging path of change, improvement, and health? Decide now, this moment, to make the choice to change. Change for the better, to walk a path you have never walked, a higher path, to see life in a new way, as an opportunity for growth, an opportunity to choose happiness, joy, and peace regardless of what passes through the door of circumstance. Be the master of your life. The master in life is the person that masters the principles of health, happiness, joy, and peace. Go back now, and choose at least one step that you know you can begin to integrate into your life. Then go forward with vigor and enthusiasm. As you begin to apply these steps to your life, you will begin to see things in a new light, a light that will reveal greater vision, truth, and possibility. If you do not do anything differently than you have always done, you will keep getting what you have always gotten. Choose now to act. Choose now so you will continually be empowered to choose in the future.

Everything you have wanted in life is possible. Choose to integrate, as you can, the steps in the preceding chapters, and you will be closer than ever before to fulfilling your dreams of health, peace, abundance, and joy in life for you and your children.

To see your child through the Eyes of Delight is the greatest gift in the world you can give to your child and to yourself.
— John Breeding